HEALTH CARE POLICY IN THE UNITED STATES

edited by

JOHN G. BRUHN
PENNSYLVANIA STATE
UNIVERSITY-HARRISBURG

A GARLAND SERIES

Health Care Policy in the United States
John G. Bruhn, editor

TELEMEDICINE IN HOSPITALS

ISSUES IN IMPLEMENTATION

SHERRY EMERY

GARLAND PUBLISHING, INC.
A MEMBER OF THE TAYLOR & FRANCIS GROUP
NEW YORK & LONDON / 1998

Library of Congress Cataloging-in-Publication Data

Emery, Sherry.
    Telemedicine in hospitals : issues in implementation / Sherry
Emery.
        p.   cm. — (Health care policy in the United States)
    Includes bibliographical references and index.
    ISBN 0-8153-3223-8 (alk. paper)
    1. Rural health services—United States—Communication
systems—Planning. 2. Hospitals—United States—Communication
systems—Planning. 3. Telecommunication in medicine—United
States—Planning. I. Title. II. Series: Health care policy in the
United States (New York, N.Y.)
RA771.5.E45 1998
362.1'028—dc21

                                                                98-29436

Printed on acid-free, 250-year-life paper
Manufactured in the United States of America

Contents

Contents

Tables

Figures

Acknowledgments

I would like to acknowledge and thank the US Office of Rural Health Policy, Health Resources and Services Administration, Public Health Service, US Department of Health and Human Services, for funding this research, which was supported by Grant # CSR000002-03-0. This work benefited tremendously from the input of the many interview subjects. Without their candor and insight, the results of this study would lack meaning and depth. To each of the individuals who took the time to speak with me about this research, I am very grateful. I would like to acknowledge the Cecil G. Sheps Center for Health Services Research for the institutional support to conduct this research, and Tom Rickets for his guidance at every stage of this project. I also thank Linda Garcia, Ken Temkin, and Elizabeth McClelland for their friendship and intellectual support. Most importantly, I thank my parents and husband, Marc Garfinkel, for their confidence and unwavering emotional support. Finally, I alone am responsible for any errors or omissions contained in this document.

Abbreviations

AHA	American Hospital Association
ANOVA	Analysis of Variance
ARF	Area Resource Files
CODEC	Coder-Decoder
COTH	Council of Teaching Hospitals
CT	Computerized Tomography
ECU	East Carolina University
GPA	Group Purchasing Alliance
GSAMS	Georgia State Academic and Medical System
HCFA	Health Care Finance Administration
HMO	Health Maintenance Organization
IDN	Integrated Delivery Network
IO	Investor Owned
MHS	Multi hospital system
MRI	Magnetic Resonance Image
MSA	Metropolitan Statistical Area
NFP	Not-for-profit
NIST	National Institute for Standards and Technology
NTIA	National Telecommunications and Information Administration
OMB	Office of Management and Budget
ORHP	Office of Rural Health Policy
OTA	Office of Technology Assessment

RUS	Rural Utilities Service
SMSA	Standard Metropolitan Statistical Area
UNC	University of North Carolina
UNC-CH	University of North Carolina-Chapel Hill

Symbols

f	function of
$\sum$	summation
/	divided by
L	log-odds
P	probability
ln	natural log

Telemedicine in Hospitals

CHAPTER 1

Introduction

telemedicine \tel-I-med-ͻ-sͻn\ *n* : technologies that allow for medical consultation between health care providers in geographically separate locations, ranging from telephone consultations to interactive video sessions using state-of-the-art technologies.

In 1968, Dr. Kenneth D. Bird solved a problem for Massachusetts General Hospital. The hospital had been responsible for staffing the medical station at Boston's Logan International Airport. Emergencies demanded an immediate, highly skilled response even though the expertise of a physician was rarely required. Therefore, during most of the staffed time at the medical station, the physician's time and labor were underutilized—a significant expense to the hospital and airport. In response to this problem, Dr. Bird developed a system for remote transmission of voice and images. Using this system, doctors working remotely from Massachusetts General Hospital performed physical examinations, made diagnoses, and even delivered limited treatments to ailing travelers using the airport's medical station (*New York Times*, February 16, 1991).

Dr. Bird was not the first innovator of telemedicine, but in the 1960s and early 1970s, his project was among the few that used microwave television technologies to transmit medical images and educational materials. For rural areas, these new telemedicine technologies promised to change how health care and medical education were accessed and delivered. Some of the pioneering telemedicine projects were very successful in achieving such promises. Yet, in its early applications, telemedicine failed to diffuse widely or to change health care dramatically. Now, more than 25 years later, the original telemedicine innovations are being transformed by advances in medical and telecommunications technologies. Once again, telemedicine holds promise as a partial solution to the health care crisis in many urban centers and rural areas of the United States.

Telemedicine, literally medicine across distance, has captured the attention of legislators, policy makers, scholars, and practitioners in the fields of health services, rural development, and telecommunications. Telemedicine combines two dynamic policy areas, health care and telecommunications, using emerging technologies to create imaginative solutions to previously intractable problems. The application of these technologies potentially improves access to health care in underserved areas and, by doing so, enhances prospects for economic development in these underserved communities. The combination of health care and telecommunications has potential that even the most jaded policy maker could not overlook. In fact, several states, including North Carolina, have cited telemedicine as a partial justification for public investment in telecommunications infrastructure, or "the information superhighway." (*Raleigh News & Observer*, May 11, 1993).

The increase in active telemedicine projects in the United States is evidence of its potential. In 1993, fewer than 30 active telemedicine programs existed nationally (Wyman 1994). By 1996, over 40 telemedicine linkages existed in North Carolina alone. Despite the phenomenal growth rate and the high visibility of telemedicine in the popular press and in the national policy arena, acceptance and financing of these technologies are uncertain. Doubt remains as to whether telemedicine will become an important component of health care at the turn of the millennium and whether telemedicine can fulfill the expectations that these technologies inspire.

What is different in the 1990s that would make telemedicine a more viable medical technology than it was in earlier decades? First, advances in telecommunications and medical technologies have increased the reliability, resolution, and speed of transmitting medical images between remote locations. Thus, telemedicine is simply more medically useful. Second, these same advances in telecommunications technologies are part of, and have fostered, changes in the national and global economies. Telecommunication technologies have intensified competition in many industries, including health care, by diminishing geographical barriers to competition. In concert with information systems, telecommunications has become a tool used by managed care corporations and hospital networks to establish competitive advantage (Coopers and Lybrand 1994, Neuberger 1995). As smaller, rural hospitals depend increasingly on telecommunications for survival (Size 1995), it is not difficult to imagine how telemedicine could become a component of these competitive strategies (Neuberger 1995).

Another difference in the 1990s that adds viability to telemedicine technology is the imperative to bolster rural hospitals, both financially and medically. During the 1980s, rural hospitals suffered because of sweeping changes in payment systems, a declining patient base due to rural out-migration, and declining inpatient utilization (Halpern et al. 1992, OTA 1990). State and federal policy makers, as well as some rural hospital administrators and larger hospital networks, see telemedicine as one way to increase rural access to health care, to augment the range of medical specialties available in rural areas, and to retain patients in rural hospitals safely.

The combination of dramatically improved medical efficacy, a changing health care marketplace, and a growing crisis in rural health care makes a compelling case for the resurgence of telemedicine in the 1990s. Two central questions emerge: (1) Does telemedicine improve rural health care delivery? and (2) Does telemedicine play a role in transforming the economic organization of the health care industry? These questions, in turn, prompt many subsidiary questions: What types of social and economic benefits does telemedicine offer? Who benefits from telemedicine technologies—hospitals, health care corporations, or communities? How do we account for or measure these benefits? How are benefits distributed and are costs and benefits balanced? What is the appropriate level of government involvement in promoting telemedicine adoption and its continued use?

Because we are only in the early stages of this new round of telemedicine diffusion, providing definitive answers to these questions is like shooting at a moving target. Published information that would answer these questions exists in anecdotal form, at best, and consists largely of logical deductions. As one researcher aptly explains, "The problem with telemedicine is that there is very little good information about it." (Perednia, quoted in Scott 1994).

In order to obtain the necessary information to address these issues, a mail survey was conducted of all general hospitals in North Carolina, South Carolina, and Georgia to explore (1) whether and when they adopted telemedicine, (2) the clinical purposes for using telemedicine technologies, (3) the business purposes for adopting these technologies, (4) how much money is invested in these technologies and the sources from which these funds originated, (5) the perceived barriers to adopting telemedicine, and (6) their level of experience with other information technologies. In order to create a working data base, the results from this mail survey were combined with data obtained from the American Hospital Association (AHA) *Guide to Hospitals in the U.S.* and the Area Resource Files (ARF). In addition, hospital administrators in the region were interviewed by telephone to obtain a richer understanding of individual telemedicine projects, general attitudes toward and beliefs about telemedicine, and the relationship between managed care and telemedicine.

With this information, a model of the diffusion of telemedicine was constructed. The theoretical underpinnings of the model represent a synthesis of sociology, management, and economic theories. The modeling begins with the assumption that adopting telemedicine is a result of combined, observable hospital and market characteristics. The functional relationship used in this research is as follows:

Probability of adopting telemedicine = f (hospital location, teaching status, size, ownership, affiliations, technological sophistication, competition from other hospitals, HMO penetration, and local population and per capita incomes).

The probability of adopting telemedicine is a function of hospital and market characteristics. By establishing the relationships between these characteristics and adoption, we are able to make inferences about the types of benefits telemedicine technologies offer and the strategic role of telemedicine technologies in a hospital's mission.

The research in this study represents a critical first step in understanding the many and complex policy questions that have emerged in the 1990s, the second round of telemedicine development. Using diffusion modeling techniques, this study describes and explains adoption of telemedicine technologies by hospitals in three states in the southeastern United States. The diffusion model used in this research makes it possible to predict what types of hospitals will adopt telemedicine and to relate that information to the types of benefits telemedicine confers and to whom. By examining the economic and policy context in which telemedicine is diffusing in this region, along with the characteristics of the hospitals adopting telemedicine, this research provides the foundation for understanding the role of telemedicine in the changing health care marketplace. This research is a snapshot of a dynamic process, providing feedback for current policy initiatives about the types of hospitals adopting telemedicine, their location, their experience with other information technologies, and their current status in the evolving market.

The findings from this study have important policy implications. Telemedicine holds great promise for improving the financial viability and quality of health care of rural hospitals; however, this research shows that rural areas are not realizing these benefits. Despite federal and state programs aimed at improving rural health through the use of telemedicine, rural hospitals are not adopting these technologies at the rate of their urban counterparts. At the same time, urban hospitals are finding ways to use telemedicine as a powerful marketing tool. Urban hospitals are also envisioning ways in which telemedicine will reduce hospital costs in a managed care environment by enhancing patient management and resource utilization. These findings suggest unrealized potential for public benefit from telemedicine and uncover substantial private—or internalizable—benefits from these technologies as well.

Such results imply a mismatch between the objectives of federal and state policies and the adoption and use of telemedicine technologies by hospitals. By identifying this incongruity, this research will help policy makers target their efforts to encourage telemedicine where it is most needed, to take advantage of market forces, and to evaluate the efficacy and necessity of current efforts. Furthermore, this research provides some of the first empirical data about telemedicine, forming the building blocks for future research in the field. This work also represents the first exploration into the relationship between telemedicine and managed care.

The remainder of this study is divided into seven chapters. By describing advances in telecommunications and telemedicine technologies and describing the federal and state policies directed to promoting telemedicine, chapter 2 provides the background of telemedicine in the 1990s. Chapter 2 also explains the major public policy issues surrounding the extensive government involvement in telemedicine development. Finally, it explores the complexities of the financial management of telemedicine in North Carolina. Chapter 3 provides a review of the relevant theoretical literature on technology diffusion, including sociological and economic approaches. Chapter 4 lays out the conceptual framework for the empirical research, including research hypotheses, modeling issues, specification of functional form, and operationalizing the diffusion model. Chapter 5 details the research design and methods, describing the survey and interviewing techniques. Chapter 6 presents the descriptive statistics, characterizing the data and the research setting. Chapter 7 analyzes the data, using the diffusion modeling techniques described in Chapter 4. Finally, Chapter 8 summarizes the research and identifies policy implications.

CHAPTER 2

Background and Foundation of Research

Telemedicine captures the imagination. These technologies suggest possibilities that justify state and federal policies for both the telecommunications and health care arenas. This seemingly simple connection of technology to policy initiatives raises some very complex economic and public policy issues. In this chapter, the technologies and range of telemedicine are described. The chapter identifies the federal and state programs that promote telemedicine and explains the public policy questions that telemedicine raises. This chapter discusses the difficulties of answering directly with quantitative data the public policy questions concerning the cost effects of telemedicine. To illustrate this point, this chapter describes three examples of prototypical telemedicine projects and suggests that diffusion modeling can begin to address these complex public policy issues.

2.1 Telemedicine: The range of possibilities

Telemedicine technologies represent a broad range of ideas and technological applications. Telemedicine can include relatively low-technology applications that are almost universally available. Some examples of low-technology applications include telephone calls or electronic-mail exchanges between medical practitioners in separate locations, facsimile transmission of fetal monitor outputs or electrocardiogram (EKG) printouts (Yamamoto and Wiebe 1989), and two-way radio transmission of medical information. More often, telemedicine describes the transmission of medical images between remote sites. In the case of teleradiology, telepathology, or teledermatology, telemedicine involves transmitting still-images between consulting physicians in distant locations: sending X rays, computerized tomography (CT) images, magnetic resonance images (MRIs), images of pathology slides, or digitized pictures of dermatological conditions. Other applications include using peripheral devices, such as electronic stethoscopes, otoscopes, or ophthalmoscopes, which are attached to audio and/or visual media for transmitting medical information between locations. In many cases, telemedicine refers to some combination of these applications. Using full-motion interactive video conferences, medical practitioners are conducting nearly every type of medical consultation that would take place in-person, including telepsychiatry (Preston, Brown, and Hartley 1992), neurology, rehabilitation, emergency medicine, as well as medical education. The most exciting, albeit currently least practical, telemedicine technologies use virtual reality and robotics technologies to enable surgeons to operate remotely (Satava 1993, 1995). The Department of Defense has developed technologies that allow surgeons, who are safely ensconced away from the battlefield, to operate on soldiers near the front lines of battle.

The key element, which is often the limiting factor in many rural areas (Puskin 1992, McCaughan 1995), to each of these applications is the conduit over which the medical information travels. Advances in communications technologies have brought about dramatic progress in the types of telemedicine consultations that are possible, making the technology more feasible and affordable. Narrowband media, such as the twisted-pair copper wires that still extend to many homes and businesses, are capable of carrying many types of telemedical information; however, the constraint of this technology is the length of time required to transmit information over a narrowband conduit. In the age of digitization, all information—from printed documents to voice messages to video images—can be represented as binary code, a string of zeros and ones. A facsimile image or voice message represents a substantially smaller quantity of information than contained in an X-ray or moving picture.

Advanced communications technologies, such as broadband media (fiber optics, coaxial cable, or satellites) accommodate greater quantities of information in a given increment of time. The difference between narrowband and broadband communications media is often compared to the difference between a garden hose and a fire hose: both are able to deliver the same amount of water, but delivery takes much more time with a garden hose. Thus, the recent and rapidly expanding availability of broadband media has dramatically increased the quantity and variety of medical information that can be delivered in a timely fashion.

Advances in compression technologies[1] allow narrowband media to resemble broadband technologies more closely (Witherspoon, Johnstone, and Wassem 1993). Areas with limited access to broadband technologies are often able to bridge the technological gap with compression technologies; these areas gain access to many telemedical applications without large public or private investments in telecommunications infrastructure.

During the past decade, not only have the technological possibilities burgeoned, but also the costs of telecommunications and telemedicine technologies have steadily decreased, effectively making these technologies more accessible. For example, the price of CODEC[2] units has decreased over 70% in recent years (Puskin 1992). Similarly, computer prices continue to fall steadily, and telecommunications expenses have decreased in many regions of the country as a result of the trend toward deregulation (Egan and Waverman 1991).

2.2 Government involvement in telemedicine

As a function of the interrelated trends of increased medical applications, growing access to broadband communications, and declining technology and telecommunications costs, telemedicine has evolved into a very practical means of delivering health care. Telemedicine holds particular promise for improving health care in rural areas, where distance is the barrier to delivering and accessing high-quality health care. Based on the promise these technologies offer, both federal and state governments have been active in promoting the adoption of telemedicine.

2.2.1 Federal government programs

Several departments of the federal government promote telemedicine through grant programs, including the following: the Department of Defense, the Rural Utilities Service (RUS; formerly, the Rural Electrification Administration), the Office of Rural Mental Health, the National Library of Medicine, the Health Care Financing Administration (HCFA), the Office of Rural Health Policy (ORHP), the National Institute of Standards and Technology (NIST), and the National Telecommunications and Information Administration (NTIA). Each program emphasizes a slightly different aspect of the benefits of telemedicine. For example, the focus of the ORHP grants is to improve access to quality health care in rural areas; the RUS grants emphasize rural development; and the NTIA includes telemedicine as part of an overall strategy to develop the National Information Infrastructure. The ORHP operates the largest grant program aimed specifically at telemedicine. In its 1995 budget, the ORHP allocated $7.4 million for new and ongoing telemedicine projects (Federal Register 1994).

2.2.2 State telemedicine initiatives

State involvement in telemedicine varies widely. Georgia, Texas, and Kansas have the oldest and most developed telemedicine networks and the longest history of state involvement with telemedicine development (Lipson and Henderson 1995). Since the late 1980s, Texas has participated in telemedicine planning and implementation (Lipson and Henderson 1995, Zetzman 1995). To date, however, the bulk of the monies for telemedicine in Texas and most other states has come from federal sources (Lipson and Henderson 1995). Georgia has contributed the most state-level direction and financial resources toward telemedicine projects, allocating a total of $12.5 million to telemedicine since 1989 (Georgia Statewide Academic and Medical System 1996) (chapter 6). As of 1995, 16 states reported state-level involvement with telemedicine projects (Lipson and Henderson 1995); in 1996, at the time of this study, two more states announced telemedicine projects (Telemedicine Research Center 1996).

2.2.3 Telemedicine use

A recent study by Abt Associates, Inc. reported that across the United States, 29% of 2,400 rural hospitals surveyed reported having some form of telemedicine capability. On average, these hospitals used telemedicine for 15 consultations with urban hospitals per month (AMNews 1996). This study focused exclusively on rural hospitals and was the first published information about the extent of telemedicine adoption. Unfortunately, the report provided no other information about the use of telemedicine by rural hospitals or comparison of telemedicine adoption and use by urban hospitals.

2.3 Telemedicine and public policy

For determining the economic feasibility and utility of telemedicine and the appropriate role for government as these technologies evolve and diffuse, it is first necessary to understand and, if possible, measure the theoretical benefits of telemedicine. If telemedicine technologies create public benefits, the role for government is well established. If telemedicine generates internalizable benefits, the role for government becomes less justifiable.

Several examples of how telemedicine can help overcome disadvantages faced by rural hospitals are standard in telemedicine literature; disadvantages can be attributed to market failures due to geography (Grigsby et al. 1993, Puskin 1992, Sanders and Tedesco 1993, Randall 1994). For example, telemedicine can reduce physician isolation by allowing rural practitioners to participate in distant programs for medical education (Preston, Brown, and Hartley 1992). This participation overcomes two rural health problems: (1) the disincentive, caused by professional isolation, for physicians to settle in rural areas and (2) the difficulty rural physicians face in maintaining state-of-the-art practices.

Telemedicine potentially improves rural access to specialty care, which is limited by the concentration of resources and specialty care in urban centers (Walker 1992; Preston, Brown, and Hartley 1992; Grigsby et al. 1994). Because it allows patients to be cared for in rural hospitals rather than transported to urban centers for specialty care, telemedicine may reduce health care costs (1) by eliminating transportation costs and

(2) by keeping patients in rural, and typically less expensive, hospitals. Moreover, by helping rural hospitals retain patients, telemedicine may improve the financial viability of rural hospitals (Arthur D. Little, Inc. 1992).

These two benefits have justified the involvement of both state and federal governments in promoting telemedicine and telecommunications infrastructure. In fact, improving rural health and the viability of rural hospitals through the use of telemedicine is the explicit goal of several state and federal telemedicine and telecommunications grant programs (Federal Register 1994, Lipson and Henderson 1994, Puskin 1993). To the extent that telemedicine addresses market failures, such as the unequal distribution of physicians or the creation of externalities like improved community health, the basis for government involvement is well established (Mueller 1989). Telemedicine is also suited, however, to improving the competitiveness of hospitals and, as a result, generating private benefits, which do not justify government intervention.

Telemedicine may produce internalizable benefits for hospitals using these technologies by generating cost savings and increasing market share. In a cost-based insurance environment, these savings may be, at least partially, passed through the health care system and viewed as partial externalities. In a capitated pricing environment, where hospitals enter contracts with insurers for a flat rate, such savings are directly internalizable. As one administrator interviewed for this research aptly explained, "The name of the game in managed care is keeping the patient in the right place." Cave (1995) phrases this strategy more academically, stressing the imperative in a capitated pricing environment to match the needs and location of enrollees to physician supply. If telemedicine facilitates decision making and augments expertise in rural areas without adding personnel, it can contribute to this type of efficiency (McCaughan 1995).

Telemedicine can also extend a hospital's market. Whether this is a public- or private-good-type benefit is a matter of perspective. On one hand, these technologies expand the range of specialties available in rural communities, potentially improving the quality of rural health care. On the other hand, telemedicine potentially increases the number of services a hospital is able to offer and/or increases the geographic range over which a hospital offers its services. These increases enhance the competitiveness of the hospital. In the case of a struggling rural hospital, improved competitiveness may translate to survival and to externalities, such as employment and improved health for the community. In the case of an already thriving hospital, increased competitiveness simply generates more profit (or reserves for not-for-profit institutions).

The issues of who benefits from telemedicine and how benefits manifest are clearly complex. So far, the potential public benefits from improved rural health care have dominated discussions about telemedicine and have justified the involvement of state and federal governments. But little empirical evidence exists to support or refute the assumption that the implementation and use of telemedicine produces public benefits.

2.4 Empirical documentation of telemedicine benefits

The original objectives of this research project were to collect data on hospital investments in telemedicine technologies and to analyze the effect of telemedicine technologies on the operating costs of a hospital. During the course of data collection and research, these goals were modified so that the objective became an examination of the patterns and reasons for the diffusion of telemedicine technologies.

Two factors prompted the decision to modify the objectives of the project. First, the survey revealed that telemedicine is in the very early stages of adoption. Of the 63 adopters of telemedicine in the sample, 27 (43%) reported the year of adoption. Of those hospitals, one (3.7%) reported the earliest year of adoption of any type of telemedicine technologies as 1993; 6 (22%) reported 1994 as the earliest year of adopting any type of telemedicine; 19 (70.4%) reported earliest telemedicine adoption in 1995, and 1 (3.7%) reported anticipated adoption in 1996. Telephone interviews with telemedicine adopters in North Carolina helped to complete information that the survey did not capture. These interviews confirmed what the survey had suggested: The majority of hospitals that adopted telemedicine had done so in late 1994 or during 1995. In fact, for over 35 hospitals in North Carolina that had adopted telemedicine and had been contacted or identified in phone interviews, only 1 had adopted telemedicine before 1994.

Recent adoption creates two major difficulties for determining the impact of these technologies on hospitals' operating costs. One difficulty is logistical. The survey asked for financial information as recent as fiscal year 1994, because at the time of the survey, hospitals were in the middle of fiscal year 1995. The majority of hospitals had implemented telemedicine in 1995. Other than for the handful of hospitals that had adopted in 1993 or 1994, calculating the financial impact of telemedicine was impossible. In fact, many hospitals were unable to report financial information for telemedicine investments. Of the 63 survey respondents who reported adopting telemedicine, 25 (39%) reported information about their financial investments in telemedicine over the past 5 years.[3] Valid statistical techniques require more than 25 observations for even the simplest models; therefore, the data were insufficient to make calculations of the aggregate cost effects of telemedicine. In the very early stages of technology adoption, it is difficult, if not impossible, to determine the long run or equilibrium impact of an innovation on an organization's costs (Porter 1980). Thus, even for those few early adopters, the financial information could not be considered reflective of true costs of operating telemedicine programs.

The second and more interesting reason why the cost model was abandoned is the complexity of the network and financing arrangements hospitals use to purchase and deploy these technologies. Because most telemedicine consultations are not currently reimbursed through the standard insurance channels, hospitals have little financial documentation of the costs and revenues generated by the purchase and use of these technologies. As a result, telemedicine projects are typically experimental, often funded with grant monies and treated as research and development activities.

The interorganizational linkages that telemedicine activities require complicate financial accounting. Most of the telemedicine networks in the study region are arranged in hub-and-spoke configurations. In many cases, the control of a telemedicine network is centralized at the hub, and the remote sites are unaware of the financial details of telemedicine projects. When a telemedicine project has been driven and financed in its early stages by the hub hospital, even though financial benefits exist for the outlying hospitals, telemedicine may not yet be integrated into operations sufficiently for financial records to be maintained.

Separate financial entities are often intermingled and new ones created to administer the multiple hospital relationships entailed in a telemedicine network. Financial arrangements between medical schools, hospital corporations, and physicians' practices are common components of telemedicine projects. Thus, the costs and the benefits of these technologies do not accrue to a single financial entity, even when the programs are initiated under the auspices of a single hospital. Such complexities make the accounting of cost and benefits at a macroeconomic or cross-sectional level very difficult. An examination of the financial and network arrangements of several North Carolina telemedicine projects illustrates this problem.

The first example represents a centralized model of telemedicine planning and financing. Although one entity has planned and implemented a network of telemedicine, the financial arrangements are complex: Six hospitals, a clinic, and a prison are all linked by telemedicine to East Carolina University (ECU) Medical School in Greenville, North Carolina. This example is one of the largest systems in the state and is among the pioneer telemedicine programs in the United States (Wyman 1994). ECU Medical School uses Pitt County Memorial Hospital as its hospital, but the university is an independent financial entity. ECU Medical School has obtained federal grant monies to develop and operate the telemedicine project; the project employs medical school staff. These activities all occur at Pitt County Memorial Hospital, but are not part of the financial records of the hospital, since they are administered by the medical school. Therefore, determining on initial inspection whether telemedicine has made an impact on the hospital's operating costs is impossible. To further complicate the scenario, the smaller hospitals connected to ECU Medical School have no record of the capital costs of implementing telemedicine because the medical school has administered the grant monies that have purchased the telemedicine equipment and financed the operating costs of the project.[4] Again, it is impossible to determine whether telemedicine has affected the operating costs of these hospitals.

The University of North Carolina (UNC) at Chapel Hill (UNC-CH) provides another example of the complex financial arrangements within a telemedicine network. Unlike the ECU model, the UNC-CH telemedicine network is not a centralized, coordinated effort. Similar to ECU Medical School, the UNC hospitals are separate financial entities from the UNC School of Medicine but share many resources and costs with the medical school. Between the UNC hospitals and the medical school, there are five active telemedicine linkages, four with other hospitals, and one with a pathology laboratory in western North Carolina. Each of these projects is administered by a different department within the UNC hospitals and medical school. For example, the UNC hospital operates a linkage with the emergency room at Wake Medical Center in Raleigh, North Carolina. Although UNC Memorial Hospital purchased the equipment and supports the operating costs of this linkage, the purpose of this project is resident training—a function of the medical school.[5] On the other hand, the pathology department in the medical school maintains a telemedicine connection with a pathology laboratory in Asheville, North Carolina. The pathology specimens from patients at UNC Memorial Hospital may be transmitted over this medical school linkage to the private clinic in Asheville. Each of the UNC telemedicine projects is administered independently by various programs or departments within the medical school. None of the programs is coordinated with other telemedicine projects at UNC-CH. Members of different projects are often unaware of other UNC telemedicine programs. According to one program manager, "There is no one at UNC who knows about all the telemedicine activities."[6] Each telemedicine project at UNC-CH is funded by separate grant monies, which are distributed through the individual programs or departments to the remote sites. As with the ECU Medical School projects, the remote sites are largely unaware of the capital costs of the technology although many sites share in the operating costs.

The North Carolina Baptist Hospital and Wake Forest University's Bowman-Gray School of Medicine provide yet another model of telemedicine implementation and accounting. Although this telemedicine program demonstrates the most developed system of cost accounting, the intricate financial arrangements involved with this network make assigning costs or savings very difficult. Interestingly, only one of the eight telemedicine projects at Bowman-Gray is financed with grant money. The remaining seven linkages are financially self-sustaining. Similar to the telemedicine programs at ECU and UNC, the eight telemedicine projects at North Carolina Baptist Hospital are affiliated with the Bowman-Gray Medical School. Unique to Bowman-Gray, these telemedicine projects are actually part of a separate corporate entity, Wake Forest University Physicians, which is an organization consisting of physicians from each of the clinical departments of the medical school. Through this organization, departments within the medical school submit a business plan for a proposed telemedicine project to the medical school. If the department can demonstrate that its telemedicine project will be financially viable, then the medical school will purchase the necessary equipment, and the department, through Wake Forest University Physicians, will support the telemedicine project's operating expenses.[7] Since the hospital, the medical school, and Wake Forest University Physicians are financially independent entities, it is impossible to link telemedicine investments to the hospital's operating costs.

These three university-based examples of telemedicine linkages account for over one half of the telemedicine activity in the state of North Carolina. These examples illustrate a broad range of coordination and accountability between the remote sites and the various departments within hospitals or medical schools. The lack of standardization across programs, or even of coordination within programs, is confusing and makes financial accounting of telemedicine all but impossible. However, this situation reflects the early stage of telemedicine development and diffusion rather than the success or failure of particular arrangements for managing telemedicine. Telemedicine is simply not well enough integrated into the operation of hospitals or the delivery of health care to determine how it affects costs.

Because telemedicine technologies are new and complex, examining the diffusion of technologies and the implications of diffusion patterns is more reasonable. From this information, it is possible to infer the types of social and economic benefits that telemedicine offers, who benefits from these technologies, and how these benefits are distributed. Then, policy goals can be compared to early outcomes. This result can be balanced with costs, and the role of government in developing telemedicine technologies can be assessed. The diffusion model represents a critical first step in understanding complex policy questions.

NOTES

1. Compression technologies use computer algorithms to delete redundant information in a series of related video frames, effectively reducing the volume of information necessary to transmit along any given communications medium (Hiatt et al. 1996).

2. CODECs, or coder-decoder technologies, transform "analog data into a digital bit stream (coder), and digital signals into analog data (decoder)." (Stallings 1991). Such transformation is an important component of many telemedicine technologies: voice signals and many video signals originate as analog signals, which must be translated into digital messages to efficiently use the communications media component of telemedicine.

3. Interestingly, six of the reported non-adopters supplied financial information for telemedicine investments. Phone interviews with the hospital administrators revealed that four of these six hospitals had not, in fact, adopted any form of telemedicine; therefore, the entries were mistakes. The other two non-adopters each had recently purchased telemedicine equipment but had not yet begun transmissions.

4. Personal communication, C. Coker, Chowan Hospital, November 8, 1995.

5. Personal communication, November through December 1995. Dr. Henry Hsiao, Professor of Biomedical Engineering, UNC-CH.

6. Ibid.

7. Personal communication, November 17, 1995, Ed Rouliski, Technical Director for Bowman-Gray School of Medicine.

CHAPTER 3

Review of the Diffusion Literature

This chapter examines theories of the diffusion of innovations and relates these theories to hospitals' adoption of telemedicine technologies. Most studies of the diffusion of innovations derive from one of two bodies of literature, one based in sociology and the other in economics. Everett Rogers (1962) is generally credited with authoring the seminal work in the sociological theory of diffusion. His *Diffusion of Innovations* outlined a model that is applied both to individual and organizational decisions to adopt innovations. Zvi Griliches (1957) conducted the first economic analysis of diffusion. In his study of hybrid corn adoption among farmers in the Midwest, Griliches found that factors influencing the profitability of an innovation played a central role in its diffusion.

As Kenneth Warner (1974, 440) explains, however, "Diffusion is not exclusively an economic phenomenon; nor is it purely sociological nor political. This complexity of the diffusion phenomenon should be reflected in the mix of variables which are studied, regardless of the principal orientation of the researcher." This chapter shares Warner's perspective, synthesizing economic and sociology theories into a framework for building the empirical component of this research. The value of this synthesis derives from the fact that health care in the United States is a quasi-economic industry with market and nonmarket characteristics and incentives. In order to understand the phenomenon of diffusion in this context, each theory provides its individual strengths. Furthermore, sociology and management theories of diffusion do a better job than economic diffusion theories in accounting for the ways information about an innovation is accessed and distributed within firms or hospitals. Although access to information is an important concept in general theories of economics, this concept is frequently ignored by economic theories of diffusion. Therefore, including noneconomic variables not only accounts for the complexity of the health care market, but also is quite consistent with general economic theory.

3.1 Economic theories of diffusion

Economic theories of diffusion typically examine how expected returns, market characteristics, and firm characteristics relate to the diffusion of a technology retrospectively, after the examined technology has diffused widely. The underlying assumption of these models is that diffusion can be described mathematically as a logistic function, whereby firms adopt an innovation at an accelerating rate throughout the first half of the process, after which adoption occurs at a decreasing rate (Griliches 1957). This process is illustrated by an S-shaped curve. The variables of interest are factors that influence the rate of adoption (Warner 1974).

3.1.1 Profitability

Within economics literature, the most prominent factor hypothesized to influence the rate of adoption is the actual or potential profitability of a given innovation. In its extreme presentation, the economics perspective relies entirely on measures of profitability to explain the diffusion process (Schultz 1964, cited in Dixon 1980): "[because] differences in profitability are a strong explanatory variable it is not necessary to appeal to differences in personality, education, and social environment."

Griliches (1957) identified profitability of the innovation as a function of (1) market characteristics, (2) the expected rate of acceptance of the innovation, and (3) the costs of the innovation and of marketing the innovation. To Griliches, the market characteristics of interest were on the supply side of the market for the innovation; he focused on the availability of the hybrid corn seed and the size of the market, measured in acres planted. In the context of a commodity-like agricultural product, this perspective makes sense because consumers are generally unaware of differences in the product other than price. Griliches' estimates of the costs of innovation and marketing were crude but important, because they formed the basis for making inferences about profitability. Subsequent studies of diffusion have been more successful in calculating the actual profitability of the innovation. For example, Klausen et al. (1992) explicitly calculated the difference in revenues that a change in clinical laboratory procedures would make for each organization in their data set. They were able to show that expected profits indeed influenced the adoption of the new technology.

In translating economic theory to the research of the diffusion of telemedicine technologies, relating direct measures of the profitability of telemedicine to hospitals' adoption of the technologies is difficult at best. As described chapters 2 and 8, individual hospitals themselves know little about the financial feasibility of telemedicine, or even how much they are investing in the innovations. Therefore, in order to examine profitability in the context of this research, exploring indirect measures of profitability is essential.

Building on Griliches' early work, other economists have explored whether factors other than measurable profitability influence the diffusion process. Although these studies examine factors other than profitability per se, the variables under consideration nearly uniformly relate back to profitability.

3.1.2 Characteristics of the innovation

Mansfield (1968) explored the relationship between diffusion and the size of the investment in an innovation. He proposed that innovations requiring smaller capital investments would diffuse faster. Also hypothesized to influence diffusion in Mansfield's model were factors such as the durability of an industry's capital stock, its rate of growth of sales, and its stage in the business cycle. However, these variables were relevant to the extent in which they affected profitability or size of the investment in an innovation over time (Stoneman 1983). Since telemedicine technologies range in expense but tend to be relatively large investments, in the Mansfield framework, they would be predicted to diffuse slowly. Although Mansfield distinguishes between the effects of profitability and the size of the investment on diffusion, it could be argued that the influence of the size of the investment on diffusion is actually another facet of profitability. To the extent that a larger investment represents a larger risk, profitability varies with the size of the investment.

3.1.3 Market structure

Several economists have explored the extent to which market structure influences diffusion, but little consensus has emerged from this research. Nelson et al. (1967) suggest that market inefficiencies are generally responsible for slower-than-optimal diffusion rates. Thus, market imperfections, such as externalities and unmeasured risks, inhibit innovation. Romeo (1977) characterized market structure in terms of competitiveness, measured by the number of firms in the industry and the variance in the firm sizes. He found that greater competition leads to more rapid diffusion. Uterback (1974) also found this to be the case.

Davies' (1979) results directly contradict these findings, showing that diffusion occurs more quickly in industries with fewer firms. Farrell and Saloner (1987) offer a potential explanation for this outcome: In their discussion of product standards, they explain that in an environment of uncertainty, competition may stifle the adoption of an innovation (like a product standard in their example) because no one wants to risk the investment involved with being a leader, in case the technology does not pay off or catch on. Again, this characteristic ultimately relates back to profitability.

The idea that market characteristics influence the diffusion of innovations is clearly a controversial one. As Stoneman (1983, 102) notes, there is no "good *a priori* reasoning to suggest" market structure would influence the rate of diffusion. Nonetheless, the hypothesis that competition or lack of competition could affect firms' perceptions about the profitability of adopting an innovation remains intriguing, policy relevant, and persistent in the literature.

Shortell, Gillies, and Devers (1995, 131) characterize the structure of the health care industry and hospitals' markets as "in a state of hyper-turbulence." The specter of managed care and the imperative to control costs highlight the potential role of market structure on the diffusion of innovations in hospitals. Although theory does not provide clear direction in predicting how market structure would affect the adoption of telemedicine technologies, the prominence of this concept in the literature and its highlighted role in the turbulent health care industry make market structure interesting for this investigation.

3.1.4 Firm characteristics

Firm Size. Deriving from Shumpeter (1969), social scientists generally hypothesize that firm size is positively related to adoption (Kimberly and Evanisko 1981, Rose and Joskow 1990). This relationship is often attributed to economies of scale, "which enhance the feasibility of adoption" (Kimberly and Evanisko 1981). Kimberly and Evanisko further elaborate the role of firm size, distinguishing between the case when size "creates a critical mass, which justifies the acquisition of particular innovations." They argue that in such a case, size facilitates adoption. In contrast, larger size necessitates the adoption of certain categories of technology, and the organization has little choice but to adopt a technology. For example, increasing size makes certain administrative innovations imperative. It can hardly be argued at this early stage of telemedicine adoption that this technology is a necessity. Rather, telemedicine would fall into the category of technologies where size is hypothesized to facilitate adoption.

In discussing the relationship between size and adoption, Rose and Joskow (1990, 354) explain that size may be a proxy for "factors such as risk aversion, participation in research and development activities, or economies of scale." In the context of telemedicine, this proposition makes sense. For smaller hospitals, the risk of a large investment in an unproven technology is much greater; thus, smaller hospitals may appear more risk averse than larger hospitals. Also, larger hospitals are more likely to have the personnel and resources to investigate and experiment with telemedicine. To the extent that the large expense is offset by higher patient volumes, economies of scale may be very relevant for telemedicine adoption.

Location. Many economic diffusion models incorporate variables denoting the geographic location of the organization as a predictor of adoption. The inclusion of location variables derives from location theory. This theory holds that characteristics of urban areas, such as agglomeration economies and dense social and economic networks, are conducive to economic growth (Isard 1956, Jacobs 1984, Maleki 1991). These concepts of generalized economic growth also apply to the specific cases of the diffusion of innovations: The agglomeration economies that provide labor and markets for growth may offer skilled labor and sufficient demand to support innovation. With respect to telemedicine, urban location could be an important variable if access to the expertise and information necessary to implement these complex technologies is correlated with geography.

Teaching status. Given that the mission of teaching hospitals may be different from the mission of other hospitals, it is plausible that the adoption behavior of teaching hospitals would be different from other hospitals. Therefore, this firm characteristic may be somewhat specific to the analysis of the diffusion of innovations in hospitals. Even though the literature does not provide predictions about the direction of this effect, the concept is uniformly represented in studies of diffusion across hospitals.

Ownership structure. Rose and Joskow (1990, 358) hypothesize that, in the electric utility industry, ownership status may affect the probability of adopting an innovation, but state "the direction of the predicted effect is ambiguous." More than electric utilities, and in fact more than most industries, the ownership structure of hospitals varies. More than one half of the hospitals in the United States are owned by not-for-profit entities (Hoerger 1991). These entities range from local municipalities and counties, to states, branches of the military and the United States government, to charitable organizations, such as churches or other religious orders. The remaining hospitals are investor-owned, for-profit institutions. Differences in ownership structure are hypothesized to influence hospitals' decisions to adopt an innovation. In line with this analysis, most studies of diffusion in hospital settings include a variable to account for ownership status.

3.1.5 Summary of economic diffusion concepts

In summary, profitability is at the heart of economic diffusion models. Detailed financial data are often proprietary or unknowable. As a result, calculations of actual or expected profits generated from a particular innovation in individual organizations are often impossible. Thus, economists have identified many factors to serve as proxies in diffusion models; these factors relate closely to profitability or have predictable influences on profitability. Market characteristics, firm characteristics, and characteristics of the innovation under investigation are standard components of economic diffusion models.

3.2 Applied models of economic diffusion

This section describes two economic studies of the diffusion of innovations in hospital settings. It is useful to examine the examples of how these researchers operationalized the theoretical economic concepts identified in the literature and to compare their results to theory.

Sloan et al. (1986) provide an example of economic theory operationalized in an analysis of hospitals' adoption of various surgical innovations. Table 3-1 summarizes the variables and concepts used in that study.

Table 3-1. A Model of the Diffusion of Surgical Techniques*

Variable	Concept
Dependent Variables: Hip arthroplasty Coronary bypass surgery Morbid obesity surgery Retina repair Cataract surgery Volume of hip arthroplasties Volume of coronary bypass	Whether the hospital has adopted one of five surgical techniques in each of 10 years in the interval between 1971 and 1981 *(categorical and time series)* Volume of cases per year *(continuous)*
Demographic Variables: Per capita income % White County 20,000–40,000 population County 40,000+ SMSA <500,000 SMSA 500,000–999,000 SMSA 1,000,000+	**Market Characteristics: Demand Side** Income and race characteristics of SMSA† of hospital or of county for non-metro hospitals. *(continuous)* Population of SMSA or county *(categorical)*

Insurance Variables: Proportion of patients that are insured by Self-pay Medicaid Medicare Blue Cross Other insurance	Payer-mix in hospital's region; influences price of hospital services: high self-pay and Medicaid ratio would drive down prices, while more privately insured patients would drive up prices. These are proxies for potential return stream associated with procedure, therefore proxies for profitability of procedure. *(continuous)*
Competitiveness of Local Market: Ratio of beds in other community hospitals to community population Mature rate setting *Availability of Complementary* *Services:* MD availability in the surgical specialty MD availability in related specialties Age of surgical specialists	**Market Characteristics: Supply Side** *(continuous)* Whether the hospital is in a region where there has been mandatory rate setting for the procedure for 2 or more years. *(categorical)* *(categorical)* *(categorical)* *(categorical)*
Hospital Characteristics: Bed size 100–249 Bed size 250–399 Bed size 400–499 Bed size 500+ Limited teaching hospital Medical school hospital COTH‡ hospital Resource need index Government hospital Proprietary hospital	**Characteristics of the Firm** Size of hospital *(categorical)* Level of medical education *(categorical)* Internal demand for the innovation; Based on case mix *(continuous)* Ownership structure: government, investor owned, or proprietary (the omitted category) *(categorical)*

†SMSA: Standard metropolitan statistical area
‡COTH: Council of Teaching Hospitals

Table 3-1 merits some explanation. Sloan et al. model the probability of a hospital adopting a given surgical technique at any given time as a function of characteristics of the hospital itself and its market. The demographic variables describe the income, race, and population characteristics of the potential demand in hospitals' markets. The insurance variables describe the payer-mix typical of the market in which a hospital operates; this is a proxy for the expected revenue stream from the surgical procedure under consideration. Together, the demographic and insurance variables describe the potential demand factors that would influence a hospital's decision to adopt the surgical innovation. On the supply side of the market transaction, Sloan et al. model adoption as a function of the competitiveness of the local market and the availability of complementary services in the community. Consistent with the economic diffusion theory, this model incorporates characteristics of the hospital, including size, teaching status, and ownership structure. An added variable is the resource need index, which measures the case mix of the hospital. This variable accounts for how relevant the innovation under consideration would be for a particular hospital, depending on the types of patients (cases) it typically provides care for.

Based on the tests of this empirical specification, Sloan et al. (1986) conclude that expected revenues (based on payer-mix) have a small, but significant and positive, effect on adoption. Similarly, higher incomes, percentage white populations, and larger size of community were positively correlated with adoption. This correlation would also indicate that greater potential income from patients positively influences adoption. The role of competition in the local market was ambiguous, but the availability of complementary services was positive and significant. Larger hospitals were much more likely to adopt the technologies, as were teaching hospitals; the effect of ownership structure was indeterminate.

For the purposes of comparison, examining another applied economic model of the diffusion of an innovation in hospitals is valuable. Tepelensky et al., (1994) test alternative models of diffusion by incorporating the respective sets of variables from three separate models into one model. In doing so, they attempt to explain the diffusion of magnetic resonance imaging (MRI) technologies. The majority of their data come from a two-staged telephone survey of hospital executives at over 500 hospitals. Table 3-2 summarizes the variables considered in their model.

Table 3-2. Hospital Adoption of Medical Technology: An Empirical Test of Alternative Models*

Variable	Concept
Dependent Variable: Adoption Date of MRI	*(categorical)* *Cross-section/time series*
CEO's Expectations: NETREV UNITAMT PREPAMT REIMB2A REIMB2B PPS PRICE	**Expected Profitability** Anticipated potential of MRI to enhance net revenues *(categorical)* Whether cost of MRI influenced adoption decision *(categorical)* Whether the cost of preparing the site for MRI influenced adoption decision *(categorical)* Whether the level of reimbursement was a positive or negative factor in adoption decision *(categorical)* Concern about prospective payment systems (DRGs, capitated pricing) *(categorical)* Anticipated influence of MRI on hospital's ability to be price competitive *(categorical)*

Competition in	**Market Characteristics: Supply Side**
Local Market:	Number of hospitals in SMSA *(continuous)*
HOSPS2	Hospitals in SMSA per 1000 people *(continuous)*
PCHOSP	SMSA Population *(continuous)*
POP1980A	Number of local competitors *(continuous)*
LOCOMP	Number of non-local competitors *(continuous)*
NOLOCOMP	Level of competition in market area for inpatient care
INPCOMP	*(categorical)*
OUTCOMP	Level of competition in market area for outpatient care
Degree of	*(categorical)*
Regulation:	Whether a Certificate Of Need (CON) was required
CONREQ	for MRIs *(categorical)*
CONDIFFH	Difficulty of CON approval for hosp-based MRIs
CONDIFFN	*(categorical)*
CONREG	Difficulty of CON approval for non-hosp MRIs
CONSCORE	*(categorical)*
RATEREG	Difficulty of CON approval for MRIs *(categorical)*
	CON stringency overall *(categorical)*
	Extent of state rate regulation *(categorical)*
Hospital	**Characteristics of the Firm**
Characteristics:	Average number of beds in hospital between 1983 and
BSC1	1986, broken down into six categories *(categorical)*
TEACHOSP	Member of Council of Teaching Hospitals
RESTRUC	*(categorical)*
HOSPKIND	Whether the hospital had been restructured in prior 3
HMARGIN	yrs *(categorical)*
MOREBEDS	Type of hospital: national or regional referral center
SEVERITY	*(categorical)*
CLINTYPE	Hospital operating margin
CDELSTRA	Whether the hospital had experienced an increase in
	the number of acute care beds *(categorical)*
	Severity of case mix *(categorical)*
	Characterization as emphasizing services that draw
	heavily on MRI
	(categorical)
	Characterization of current service delivery strategy as
	being unchanging *(categorical)*

Perception of	**Characteristics of the Management**
Risk:	Concern about early obsolescence of MRI technology
OBSOLETE1	*(categorical)*
UNCUNIT1	Uncertainty about type of MRI to purchase/lease
UNCMAG1	*(categorical)*
PROVCLIN	Uncertainty about magnet size and type of MRI
POTCLIN	*(categorical)*
CAPITAL	Influence of proven clinical applications on adoption
Strategic	*(categorical)*
Importance of	Influence of potential clinical applications on adoption
Technology:	*(categorical)*
TECHDEV	Whether the availability of capital influenced the
DEVSTRAT	adoption decision *(categorical)*
TECHTYPE	Importance of being perceived as a technology leader
PRICEDEV	in a hospital's market development strategy
Level of	*(categorical)*
Decision	Most important market development strategy is being
Making:	perceived as technology leader *(categorical)*
IDEA1	Emphasis on high tech products, programs, or services
INVOLVE	*(categorical)*
CFOMRI	Importance of being price competitive to hospital's
	strategy *(categorical)*
	Source of idea to acquire MRI (administration or
	medical staff)*(categorical)*
	High involvement by medical staff in decision to
	adopt MRI *(categorical)*
	Strong CFO involvement in decision making
	(categorical)

Tepelensky et al. (1994) model the diffusion of MRI as a function of several measures of expected profitability, market characteristics (including measures of competitiveness and regulation), characteristics of the management (orientation toward the technology), and the strategic role of the technology in the hospital. The object of their study was to test the significance of the strategy variables to determine whether the predominant reason for adopting a technology in a hospital setting is profit maximization, technological preeminence, or clinical excellence. They identify the other variables accounting for market and organizational characteristics as control variables. The study shows that (1) hospitals emphasizing the strategy of technological leadership are significantly more likely to adopt MRI technology, (2) larger hospitals are more likely to adopt, (3) regulation inhibits adoption, (4) the expectation that the technology will increase revenue improves the odds of adoption, (5) involvement of the medical staff in the decision increases the odds of adoption, and (6) involvement of the chief financial officer (CFO) reduces the odds of adoption. These findings provide qualified support for the economic theory of diffusion. In this study, technological leadership—a form of nonprice competition—was quite a powerful predictor of adoption, whereas financial variables were less important. However, the fact that CFO involvement may reduce the probability of adoption may indicate that, in cases where financial concerns are prominent, the technology is less attractive. This study is interesting because it incorporated variables and concepts that account for management style and explicit statements of hospital strategy. As such, it helps explore the adequacy of the assumption that profit drives the adoption of innovations in hospital settings.

3.3 Noneconomic theories of diffusion

This section briefly discusses models of the diffusion of innovations that derive from entirely different theoretical perspectives. In some cases, economists and sociologists or management theorists use different language to discuss very similar ideas. In many instances, however, the perspective of other branches of social science differ from economics quite a bit.

3.3.1 Rogers' theory of diffusion

Nearly every noneconomic study (and several economic studies) of the diffusion of innovations refers to Everett Rogers' *Diffusion of Innovations*, first published in 1962. In Rogers' framework, the process of adopting an innovation occurs in five stages. First, the potential adopter becomes aware of, or gains *knowledge* about the innovation. Next comes *persuasion*, when the potential adopter forms a positive or negative opinion about the innovation. Formation of an opinion leads to the *decision* whether or not to adopt. Decision making is followed by *implementation*, when the innovation is put into use, and *confirmation* of the utility of the innovation:

Knowledge ➔ Persuasion ➔ Decision ➔ Implementation ➔ Confirmation

For each stage, the following features are of interest: characteristics of the potential adopter, characteristics of how information about the innovation is communicated, and characteristics of the innovation itself. For example, how does an individual or organization obtain knowledge about an innovation? What are the reasons for seeking such knowledge? What characteristics of individuals or organizations are associated with knowledge-seeking behavior or receptivity to knowledge about innovations? After knowledge is obtained, what characteristics of the innovation, the channel of communication about the innovation, and the potential adopter are related to forming a positive opinion of the innovation?

Classical theories of diffusion identify individual characteristics that are associated with receptivity to and adoption of innovations (Greer 1977). Some of these characteristics include age, as well as being cosmopolitan, liberal, and prestige-seeking. In an organizational context, classical sociological studies identify factors including organizational complexity, locus of decision making, and size as important predictors of innovative behavior (Baldridge and Burnham 1975, Greer 1977).

Whereas economists identify factors related to profitability as being the strongest form of persuasion to adopt an innovation, sociologists use different concepts. For example, the language used by McKinney et al. (1991, 19) to describe how a hospital characteristic might affect adoption illustrates the differences between the economic and the sociological approaches: "membership in a multihospital system or alliance should provide the *social legitimation* and technical support necessary to accomplish implementation" (emphasis added). The key differences between sociology- and economics-based approaches are the factors that are assumed to be constant across observations. For economists, all individuals and organizations are rational economic entities, whose behavior is neither idiosyncratic nor determined by variables other than economic considerations. For sociologists, factors, such as profitability and access to capital, are invariant across individuals or organizations whose behavior is determined by unique characteristics and experiences. While both theory bases include characteristics of the organization and innovation in their models, these variables represent very different concepts.

For the purpose of this research, two sociological concepts are important in modeling diffusion: (1) the role of experience with or exposure to an innovation and (2) communication about an innovation. While economic theory often refers to situations of perfect information, or market failures resulting from imperfect information, this concept is absent from economic diffusion models. As Rogers (1983) points out, an individual's exposure to an idea is instrumental to their obtaining knowledge—or information—about that idea or innovation. Since knowledge is the precursor to subsequent diffusion events, this exposure is critical. In economic terms, Rogers' theory accounts for differential access to information about an innovation. In the context of telemedicine adoption, exposure to or experience with other information technologies (such as hospital information systems) may be sufficiently similar to lay the groundwork for obtaining knowledge and forming opinions about telemedicine technologies.

Sociology-based models of diffusion also explore the access to, complexity of, and individual relationships to channels of communication about innovations (Greer 1977, Fennel and Warnecke 1988). In a very concrete, hospital-based example, McKinney et al. (1991, 17) cite Kimberly (1987), explaining that "because these systems and alliances build linkages between local hospitals, regional offices, and corporate headquarters, they have the potential to function as 'innovation carriers', " accelerating the diffusion of innovations. Thus, in economic terms, membership in these networks represents a form of potentially asymmetric information. Following such reasoning and applying it to economic concepts of the role of information in markets, the research presented in this study will incorporate the sociological concept of communication networks into the economic modeling of diffusion. In the following chapter, these theoretical constructs are applied to the diffusion of telemedicine technologies in hospitals.

CHAPTER 4
Conceptual Framework

In this chapter, the conceptual framework that guided the empirical research is specified. The chapter first identifies the research hypotheses and the variables of interest, then utilizes economic diffusion theory to provide a theoretical framework for the empirical analysis. As part of this task, the section explains and justifies the functional form of the diffusion model. Finally, the chapter describes the data necessary to carry out the research, operationalizes the critical variables, and identifies data sources.

As explained in chapter 3, economic theory holds that firms—in this case, hospitals—will adopt a technology if the benefits exceed the costs. In the absence of market imperfections, such as differential access to information or capital, economic theory predicts that larger, urban organizations will be more likely to adopt an innovation. Additional factors, such as competitiveness of the local market, ownership structure, and other hospital characteristics, are important, but the direction of their influence is uncertain. In the context of this research, such factors are of particular interest because they help determine the appropriate role for government in the financing and diffusion of telemedicine.

Oftentimes, direct measures of profitability are unavailable, and characteristics of the innovation or the firm are used as proxies or alternative measures of potential profitability. This situation is certainly the case for telemedicine; in many cases, hospitals themselves do not yet know whether these technologies will be profitable.

4.1 Research hypotheses

In this research, three primary hypotheses are proposed. Two of the primary hypotheses have subsidiary hypotheses, which further explore the relationships posed in the primary hypotheses. Not every hypothesis or subsidiary holds equal weight in terms of policy-relevance or general interest. Nonetheless, each is important in exploring and explaining the interrelated phenomena involved with adoption and use of telemedicine technologies. Each hypothesis and its subsidiaries will be discussed in the context of its policy and/or theoretical motivation. The first hypothesis (H1) follows:

H1. Urban hospitals are more likely to adopt telemedicine technologies. From a policy perspective, this is an important hypothesis because it tests the match between policy goals and early outcomes; it also provides evidence about the current status of the public benefits that justify many government telemedicine policies. This hypothesis is controversial, given that legislators, policy makers, the popular press, and the community of telemedicine scholars identify telemedicine with rural health.

Expecting that urban hospitals would be more likely to adopt telemedicine technologies than rural hospitals is reasonable. A prominent theory, which is presented in the economic literature along with several studies of the diffusion of other industrial and medical technologies, suggests that rural communities lack the constellation of factors that would make adopting telemedicine feasible or affordable (Isard 1956, Jacobs 1984, Maleki 1991). This constellation includes sufficient demand for medical services, adequate or affordable telecommunications infrastructure, and the expertise or slack resources to study and implement telemedicine. Moreover, to the extent that these technologies are typically quite expensive and are lumpy goods—where a threshold investment is necessary before the technologies can be useful—rural hospitals often do not have the financial resources necessary to adopt telemedicine. Nor do rural hospitals typically have management resources, in terms of time, experience with technology, or personnel, to investigate and implement these technologies. Thus, urban or rural status measures not only a geographic influence, but serves as a proxy for other hospital attributes. Despite the fact that geography alone would suggest that these technologies would be most useful to rural hospitals, other factors associated with rural location suggest that urban hospitals would be more likely to adopt telemedicine. Hypothesis 1 is tested using a logistic regression equation, modeling the probability of adopting telemedicine as a function of characteristics of the hospital, including rural status.

H1a. Hospital size is positively related to telemedicine adoption. As a subsidiary to the first hypothesis, larger hospitals are expected to be more likely to adopt telemedicine than smaller hospitals. This hypothesis is less policy-relevant than the associated primary hypothesis. However, it identifies one factor that is highly correlated with rural location, but the factor may exert an independent influence on telemedicine adoption. Therefore, testing for an association between the variables representing size and geographic location is important, along with determining which variable is a more important predictor of adoption, if such association exists.

The expectation that larger hospitals are more likely to adopt telemedicine is based on much of the same reasoning as used for the primary hypothesis: Larger hospitals typically have greater financial and managerial resources than smaller hospitals. As a result, important economies of scale may exist in terms of telemedicine adoption. If substantiated, this finding would provide vital information to help policy makers better tailor their programs to reach the hospitals with most need.

H1b. Management sophistication with regard to technology is positively related to telemedicine adoption. As with hypothesis H1a, the importance of this hypothesis lies in its potential to unravel the complex factors represented by rural location. On the basis of innovation diffusion theory and common sense, this hypothesis predicts that hospitals with greater sophistication for managing technology are more likely to adopt a very technical innovation like telemedicine (Rogers 1983). If this research demonstrates an association between technological sophistication and telemedicine adoption, it would again provide fundamental information that would allow policy makers to better target their programs.

H2. Ownership structure is a factor in the adoption of telemedicine. This hypothesis helps identify the types of benefits hospitals may obtain from telemedicine. As the types of benefits are identified, the appropriate role for government would be better defined. If investor-owned (IO) and not-for-profit (NFP) hospitals have different patterns of adoption, it is reasonable to infer that the benefits offered by telemedicine may be more important to one group than the other.

Economic theory provides little guidance about how ownership structure would affect a hospital's behavior, other than to suggest that IO and NFP hospitals may behave differently (Arrow 1963, Alexander and Lewis 1984, Hoerger 1991, Sear 1991). The theory proposes that IO hospitals may have more narrowly defined objective functions (i.e., organizational goals) since they are accountable to shareholders and therefore more subject to profit maximization requirements than NFP hospitals. By this reasoning, NFP hospitals theoretically have broader missions, such as serving indigent populations or providing other community services, which make profit maximization a lower priority. Even this proposition is controversial. Several studies have demonstrated no difference between IO and NFP hospitals in community service orientation, efficiency, or profitability (Sloan and Vraciu 1983, Friedman and Shortell 1988, Kralewski and Gifford 1988).

Some factors specific to telemedicine technologies would suggest that IO and NFP hospitals may differentially adopt telemedicine. First, federal and state governments have played a strong role in promoting the development of these technologies through grant programs, such as those described in chapter 2. In many cases, IO institutions may not be eligible for these types of funding. To the extent that grant monies provide the added incentive for hospitals to adopt telemedicine when they otherwise would not, NFP hospitals would be more likely to adopt telemedicine than IO hospitals, which are unable to take advantage of such incentives.

Second, to the extent that IO and NFP hospitals do face different objective functions, their attitudes about telemedicine and their behavior regarding telemedicine adoption may vary. The policy implications of this hypothesis are important. If IO hospitals adopt telemedicine at least as readily as NFP hospitals, it could be argued that the benefits of these technologies are largely internalizable. In this scenario, there is little justification for government involvement. In contrast, if NFP hospitals are more likely than IO hospitals to adopt telemedicine, several inferences could be drawn. First, it is possible that government programs are successfully encouraging the diffusion of telemedicine in hospitals eligible for state and federal funds. Second, telemedicine may not be a profitable investment and thus requires government involvement in order to stimulate adoption. Third, telemedicine may play a role in the broader missions of NFP hospitals, objectives that are not shared by IO hospitals. None of these inferences is necessarily a direct consequence of a difference in behavior, which the diffusion model would identify. If such a difference is apparent, it identifies a need to further explore the differences between IO and NFP hospitals that would lead to this outcome.

The test of this hypothesis is very straightforward: A dummy variable, indicating ownership structure, is included in the logit model. If this variable is statistically significant, ownership structure cannot be ruled out as a factor influencing the adoption of telemedicine.

H3. Telemedicine is an important technology for hospitals anticipating changes, specifically managed care, in the health care marketplace. The third primary hypothesis examines the role that telemedicine plays in hospitals' strategies to adapt to managed care. This hypothesis is very important from a policy perspective because it examines the intersection of public policies, which are motivated by the need to provide a public-good, with turbulent market forces.

Telemedicine technologies have been slow to diffuse in markets where managed care has significant penetration. On the basis of this observation, it is likely that this hypothesis would be rejected. However, managed care is most evolved in cities such as Los Angeles, California; San Diego, California; Minneapolis, Minnesota; St. Paul, Minnesota; and Worcester, Massachusetts (Hospitals & Health Networks 1995). Among other factors, these cities all have in common a density of population, health care providers, and hospitals that provide geographically concentrated market competition (Curran and O'Connor 1995; Kripke Byers and Levi-Baumgarten 1995). In the Southeast, such density does not exist. Telemedicine potentially extends the geographic reach of hospitals' markets; thus, telemedicine could be an important tool in simulating the density of patients and health care providers that exists in more evolved managed care markets. Therefore, managed care may be an important impetus to adopting telemedicine in the southeastern United States.

Hypothesis 3 also probes the effect that alternative arrangements for medical financing may have on the diffusion of telemedicine. Currently, third-party insurers do not reimburse hospitals or physicians for most telemedicine consultations. In the absence of subsidization, telemedicine is not a financially attractive endeavor, unless it contributes to savings, which could be internalized under a capitated pricing scheme common to many managed care plans. Consequently, telemedicine could be an important tool not only to improve market share, but also to create internalizable benefits in a managed care environment.

The policy implications of this hypothesis are numerous and important. If telemedicine is, in fact, a strategic technology that hospitals adopt in response to or in anticipation of competitive pressures, the role of state and federal governments in promoting these technologies comes into question: (1) Are government inducements to encourage telemedicine adoption necessary? (2) Do these federal and state projects help all hospitals that receive funds supporting telemedicine to become more competitive? (3) Are the hospitals most in need of assistance to become viable or competitive in a changing marketplace adopting telemedicine and/or benefiting from federal or state aid?

By testing hypothesis 3, it is possible to determine the relevancy and answers to the corollary questions. The tests of hypothesis 3 are threefold. First, a variable measuring actual competition in the hospitals' local market is incorporated into the diffusion model. While this test does not directly address the managed care question, it provides information about local competitive pressures faced by hospitals. Second, descriptive statistics are used to analyze the answers of telemedicine adopters to Likert scale questions, which ask how important telemedicine technologies are to their managed care strategy. Third, qualitative information obtained in interviews with hospital administrators and directors of telemedicine projects supplements the quantitative evidence, providing supporting or contradictory evidence of the quantitative results. The tests of the subsidiary hypotheses also help to probe hypothesis 3.

H3a. Affiliation with other hospitals or health care organizations is positively related to telemedicine adoption. This hypothesis is important from several policy perspectives. As described, the health care markets in the southeastern United States have not evolved very far along the continuum between unstructured markets and high penetration of managed care. A significant step in this evolution is forming strategic alliances among hospitals (Cave 1995; Curran and O'Connor 1995; Hospitals and Health Networks 1995; Kripke Byers and Levi-Baumgarten 1995; Nurkin 1995; Shortell, Gillies, and Devers 1995). Therefore, telemedicine technologies are expected to play a role in strategic alliances if they are part of a strategy for preparing for managed care. Moreover, the literature in innovation diffusion in hospitals suggests that membership in such alliances is associated with the adoption of new technologies or innovations (McKinney, Kaluzny, and Zuckerman 1991). As such, this subsidiary to hypothesis 3 helps to elucidate the relationship proposed in the primary hypothesis.

Hospital alliances have been the subject of considerable interest to the Justice Department and the Federal Trade Commission (AMNews 1996). As hospital networks grow, so do concerns about antitrust issues. To the extent that telemedicine both depends on and facilitates linkages between hospitals, it could be at the center of a very controversial policy debate.

Alliances can take several forms (Moscovice et al. 1991; Zuckerman, Kaluzny, and Ricketts 1995). The hypothesis that membership in a strategic alliance is a factor in telemedicine adoption is tested by including alliance variables in the logistic regression model predicting the adoption of telemedicine. These variables represent three forms of alliances: membership in a multihospital system, membership in a group purchasing alliance, and membership in an integrated delivery network.

H3b. The degree of penetration by health maintenance organizations in a hospital's market is positively related to telemedicine adoption. This hypothesis explores whether a relationship currently exists between the adoption of telemedicine and the concurrent trend of growing market forces, represented by the growth in health maintenance organization (HMO) enrollment. If telemedicine is a competitive tool, as suggested, we would expect that higher HMO penetration would be related to the adoption of telemedicine. This hypothesis is difficult to test in the Southeast, where HMO penetration is generally low relative to other regions of the United States. Nonetheless, variation exists within the region and between urban and rural areas. Hypothesis 3b is tested in two ways. First, a variable measuring HMO penetration in the hospital's county or metropolitan statistical area (MSA) is included in the logistic regression equation. Again, in testing this hypothesis, checking and controlling for association with the urban/rural variable is important. Second, hospital administrators and telemedicine project managers were interviewed to ascertain whether and to what extent telemedicine played a role in the managed care strategies of their hospitals.

4.2 Modeling the problem

This section presents the development of the model that explains the adoption of telemedicine technologies by hospitals. A synthesis of economic, sociology, and management theories provide the theoretical framework for the model of technology adoption. The value of this synthesis derives from the fact that health care in the United States is a quasi-economic industry with market and nonmarket characteristics and incentives. For example, some hospitals are investor-owned (IO) businesses and, as such, are considered for-profit institutions. Consequently, they are assumed to conform to the profit-maximization assumptions of an economic diffusion model. Other hospitals are not-for-profit (NFP) institutions, owned and controlled by churches or governments.[1] While it is reasonable to assume that for-profit and not-for profit hospitals behave differently (Arrow 1963, Hoerger 1991), there are equally compelling reasons to assume similar behavior. Many theories of the objective function of NFP hospitals exist (Arrow 1963, Newhouse 1970, Lee 1971, Pauly and Redisch 1973), but it is difficult to show empirically a difference in behavior between IO and NFP hospitals because it is "impossible to observe a hospital's utility function, or even its maximum possible profit"[2] (Hoerger 1991). Moreover, because IO and NFP hospitals compete in the same marketplace, it is reasonable to assume that their behavior would not differ significantly, even if they face different objective functions. This project begins with the assumption that all hospitals behave, more or less, as profit maximizers, and therefore can be characterized by an economic model.

The model-building component of this research also reflects the fact that many of the variables included in economic models of diffusion are included in sociological diffusion models. Of these variables, many have no economic interpretation, per se, but improve the explanatory power of the models. Because these variables figure prominently in both theory bases and because they can explain the behavior of hospitals, they are included in the framework used in this research.

4.2.1 Identifying the dependent variable

Whether a hospital had adopted telemedicine by the end of fiscal year 1995 is represented as a binary dependent variable. It would be ideal to identify more specifically how a hospital intends to use the telemedicine technologies it has chosen to adopt. For example, some hospitals serve exclusively as providers of telemedicine consultations; in contrast, other hospitals primarily receive consultations. Conceivably, some hospitals would serve as both providers and receivers of telemedicine consultations. Among the different categories of adopters, it is reasonable to expect that the motivations for adopting telemedicine and the characteristics of the hospitals and their markets would differ. While the econometric specification of this type of dependent variable, or polytomous response variable, is straightforward, obtaining the data to conduct this type of analysis proved problematic. The survey instrument asked hospitals to designate the volume of telemedicine consultations received and provided for a variety of applications; however, the number of hospitals that responded to this set of questions was too small to use in a statistical model. In subsequent telephone interviews, several hospital administrators indicated that their telemedicine programs were so young that they were not yet tracking this type of information. Using telephone interviews to obtain information about which category of adoption each hospital in the study represented was prohibitively expensive in terms of both time and money. Thus, the dependent variable for this research is simply a binary variable, representing whether a hospital had adopted any form of telemedicine technology at the time of the survey. While this specification is not ideal, it is still quite useful from a policy perspective, and more importantly, represents the first empirical research on telemedicine adoption.

The approach of using a binary dependent variable contrasts with much of the economic literature, which models the time a firm takes to adopt a particular innovation as a dependent variable (Griliches 1957, 1989; Rose and Joskow 1990; Sloan et al. 1986; Stoneman 1983; Tepelensky et al. 1994). This approach, however, conforms to much of the sociology literature, which models the adoption of an innovation as a function of behavioral variables and individual characteristics (Baldridge and Burnham 1975, Greer 1977, Kimberly 1982, Fennell and Warnecke 1988).

Although telemedicine has existed for over 30 years, the diffusion process has not been continuous (Grigsby 1994). Perednia and Brown (1995) report that "fewer than ten telemedicine programs existed in the United States in 1990." In fact, over 90% of the hospitals that reported a telemedicine adoption date for this research project adopted the technologies in 1994 or 1995. Telemedicine diffusion in the 1990s, therefore, is essentially an entirely new and separate phenomenon from that of earlier decades since little to no adoption took place in the intervening period. Given the lack of variability in the date for adopting this technology, taking the more traditional diffusion modeling approach with this subject and these data would yield inconclusive results. For this reason, the diffusion model used in this project is more similar to the dependent variable of sociological models than to economic models.

4.2.2 The diffusion paradigm applied: Identifying independent variables

As explained in chapter 3, economic diffusion theory can be summarized simply: Firms will adopt a technology if they expect adoption to be profitable. This simplicity quickly becomes complex when we try to understand what factors influence these expectations and hence predict adoption. Though economists differ widely in the particular variables they choose for explaining diffusion, economic theory suggests three broad categories of relevant variables: (1) real or expected returns of innovation-investments, (2) market characteristics, and (3) firm characteristics. The first category is a direct measure of actual or expected returns from investments in an innovation; the second two categories measure indirectly the profitability of an innovation and the factors that contribute to its profitability.

Because it is so early in the diffusion of telemedicine technologies, financial data about telemedicine are virtually nonexistent. Moreover, because insurers do not yet reimburse for most telemedical consultations, the anticipated revenues from these technologies is not a predictable variable that would improve the model's explanatory powers. Therefore, this research focuses on modeling the effects of market and firm characteristics on the adoption of telemedicine.

In this research, another category of explanatory variables drawn from sociological or communications theory is added. This category consists of two types of variables measuring sociological concepts: (1) one type of variable that measures hospitals' experience with or exposure to other telecommunications and information technologies and (2) the second type, which includes three variables that account for associations with other hospitals. While all four of these behavioral variables could logically be included among hospital characteristics as one of the economic typologies, they are separated here because sociology theory provides a more robust and well-developed framework for understanding the role of these variables in an organization's decision to adopt innovations. Thus, the model in this research project uses three categories of variables to explain hospitals' adoption of telemedicine technologies:

Equation
(1) Adoption of telemedicine $= f$ (market characteristics, hospital characteristics, behavioral characteristics).

4.3 Defining the variables

This section is based on the theoretical relationships established in chapter 3 and the preceding hypotheses. It identifies the variables included in the diffusion model.

4.3.1 Market characteristics

For the purposes of this research, two aspects of market structure are relevant: (1) the degree of competitiveness on the supply side of hospital services and (2) the market for hospital services, comprising the demand side, in the form of patient-base.

The Supply Side. On the supply side, there are two important dimensions to competition. First, other hospitals represent competition in the market. Second, the level of managed care penetration is an indicator of the intensity of cost-containing pressures in the local market. What constitutes a hospital's market is an issue of significant complexity and recent controversy. Nationally recognized centers of excellence draw patients from all over the country or the world to take advantage of unique therapies, equipment, or well-known specialists in a given field. Generally, however, a hospital's market is geographically bounded (Gesler and Cromartie 1985).

Sloan et al. (1986) model competition as the ratio of beds in other community hospitals to community population. The community is defined as the hospital's metropolitan statistical area (MSA) boundary or county for nonmetropolitan hospitals. This measure is attractive because it accounts both for supply and demand. A high number of beds in other hospitals will occur in regions with high populations because such areas typically support many hospitals. By calculating the ratio of other beds per capita, Sloan et al. (1986) control for this heteroskedastic effect and relate supply to demand: A low ratio indicates little competition relative to the size of the population, and a high ratio indicates greater competition. Tepelensky et al. (1994) use similar measures of competition: the number of hospitals in the MSA and the number of hospitals per capita in the MSA. However, these measures are not as precise as those of Sloan et al. (1986) and suffer the same problems.

For regions, such as North Carolina and much of the southeastern United States, where population is relatively evenly distributed across counties or MSAs, this measure is flawed because it neglects the possibility that patients would cross county or MSA boundaries to receive hospital care.[3] An alternative measure relies on geographic definitions of a hospital's service area. The literature in medical geography provides extensive discussion about the most appropriate method of defining a hospital's service area and includes debate about the relative advantages of defining service areas by geographic distance, geopolitical boundaries, or patient origin (Simpson et al. 1994). Of these three potential referents, for the purposes of this study, the most appropriate definition of a hospital's service area would rely on geographic distance.[4] Simpson et al.

(1994, 211) explain that this technique has been used "to study competition for clients among neighboring hospitals." For the purposes of this research, competition from other hospitals is measured as the distance to the next closest hospital, an approach that follows the theory of medical geographers.

Percentage of the population in the hospital's MSA or county that is enrolled in an HMO is used as an index of managed care penetration, another supply-side market characteristic. Although it would be ideal to measure HMO enrollment within a given geographic radius of the hospital, the data do not exist in this form. The designation used here comes from the 1994 Area Resource Files (ARF) and is based on the United States Office of Management and Budget (OMB) designations of metropolitan areas, wherein all areas not included in MSAs are considered nonmetropolitan, or rural.

Another form of competition, which is not included in this telemedicine diffusion model, can be characterized as competition to telemedicine. This variable takes the form of alternatives to telemedicine that exist within the market. The availability of physician specialists within a community could be considered competition to telemedicine. On the other hand, a hospital located in a region with an abundance of specialists may adopt telemedicine in order to offer, rather than receive, consultations. Similar to defining market competition, this variable is also complicated by problems of defining relevant market boundaries. Sloan et al. (1986) used the availability of physician specialists within the hospital's MSA or county as an indicator of access to specialists. Like patients, however, physician practices do not necessarily correspond neatly with geopolitical units, particularly in the Southeast. In addition, the availability of specialists is highly correlated with urban locations. Finally, although it is theoretically possible to calculate the density of specialists within a given radius of a hospital, secondary data do not exist in this form. The lack of practical feasibility combined with ambiguous theoretical expectations about this variable make it unattractive to include in the diffusion model for this research.

The Demand Side. Measures of market population and demographic characteristics, such as income and race, are standard in the literature (Sloan et al. 1986, Tepelensky et al. 1994) on diffusion of innovations in hospitals. Following the convention in the literature, this research includes parameters of the demand side of the hospitals' markets in the diffusion model. The variables of interest are the number of potential patients in the hospital's market and their purchasing power for hospital services. The size of the patient base is measured by population in the MSA or county. It is important to test for association between this variable and the urban/rural (MSA/non-MSA) variable.

Ideally, a measure of the percentage of the population with any form of medical insurance would account for the purchasing power for hospital services in a given market. Since insurers currently do not reimburse for most telemedical consultations (Grigsby 1994), the assumption that this factor is not an important demand characteristic for telemedicine is necessary. Moreover, these data are not available. Therefore, per capita income in the MSA or county is used as a proxy for purchasing power for hospital services. Naturally, in MSAs or counties with wide ranges of personal incomes, this measure is not ideal. In fact, the average income could present a distorted picture of purchasing power in regions where very high incomes are offset by very low incomes. Nonetheless, this measure is attractive because it is convenient. The data for both demand parameters come from the ARF data set.

4.3.2 Hospital characteristics

The diffusion literature and the hypotheses specified in this research suggest four hospital characteristics to include in the model of telemedicine diffusion: (1) location, (2) teaching status, (3) size, and (4) ownership.

Whether a hospital is in an urban or rural *location* is of particular interest. Telemedicine technologies hold promise for revitalizing health care delivery in rural areas if the technologies are adopted in rural areas. For this project, a hospital is considered urban if it is situated within an MSA; conversely, a hospital is categorized as rural if it is located outside MSA boundaries. These data are available from the Area Resource Files (ARF).

Whether a hospital engages in *teaching* medical students and/or residents may affect the likelihood of adopting a technology such as telemedicine. The mission of teaching hospitals includes an orientation toward innovation. Moreover, hospitals affiliated with universities may have greater access to and experience with writing grants; grants often fund the initial investment in telemedicine. Thus, teaching hospitals are expected to be more likely to adopt telemedicine. For the purposes of this research, a hospital is considered a teaching hospital if it is a member of the Council of Teaching Hospitals. The American Hospital Association (AHA) *Guide to Hospitals in the U.S.* provides these data.

Economic diffusion theory suggests that *size* is positively correlated with the adopting an innovation (David 1969, Rose and Joskow 1990). Hospital size, which is measured by the number of licensed beds, is an important variable for this research because it closely relates to geographic location. Larger hospitals are typically located in urban areas, while smaller hospitals are most often found in rural areas. The AHA *Guide* supplies these data.

Ownership status is included in this model to test hypothesis 2. Because it is quite conceivable that investor-owned (IO) and not-for-profit (NFP) hospitals have different objective functions (Arrow 1963, Newhouse 1970, Lee 1971, Pauly and Redisch 1973), it is necessary to control and test for different behaviors in terms of adopting telemedicine technologies. For this reason, this research classifies hospitals as for-profit institutions if they are investor-owned. Hospitals are considered NFP if they are owned by local, state, or federal governments or owned by religious or other nonprofit organizations. These data come from the AHA *Guide*.

4.3.3 Behavioral characteristics

The familiarity of a hospital with other telecommunications and information technologies is considered a behavioral characteristic because sociology and communications theories present a more thoroughly developed framework about the role of knowledge of an innovation's existence and the probability of adoption. As Rogers (1983) explains, the decision whether to adopt an innovation begins with the knowledge of its existence. Because telemedicine technologies are sophisticated permutations of telecommunications and information technologies, this research posits that a manager's familiarity with information systems would correlate with a greater likelihood of knowing telemedicine exists and being receptive to such technological applications. An index of technological sophistication, constructed from the survey responses to questions about the adoption of hospital information systems, measures this concept in the model.

Finally, hypothesis 3a and sociological diffusion theory motivate the inclusion of variables that account for a hospital's *affiliations* with other hospitals as predictors of telemedicine adoption. As described, such affiliations can take many forms, but three are identified for the purposes of this research. Membership in a multihospital system (MHS), a group purchasing alliance (GPA), and an integrated delivery network (IDN) are considered. These categories are not mutually exclusive, so each is included in the model as a dummy variable. These data come from the survey undertaken as part of this research project.

Table 4-1 provides a summary of the variables included in the diffusion model and their sources.

Table 4-1. Diffusion Model Variables for Telemedicine

Variable	Concept/Type of Variable	Source
Dependent variable Q1ANEW	*(categorical)* Coded as 1 if hospital adopted Telemedicine; 0 if not.	Survey
Market Characteristics		
Competition from other hospitals NEAREST	*(continuous)* Distance to next closest hospital; a measure of competition from other hospitals.	ARF data Romeo (1977), Rose and Joskow (1990). Hypothesized effect: (?)
Managed care penetration HMOPEN	*(continuous)* Percentage of population in MSA or county enrolled in an HMO.	ARF data Hypothesized effect: (+)
Size of patient base POPULAT	*(continuous)* Population of the MSA or county (in 1000s)	ARF data Sloan et al. (1986); Tepelensky et al. (1994). Hypothesized effect: (+)
Potential ability to pay for services INCOME	*(continuous)* Per capita income of MSA or county (in 100s).	ARF data Sloan et al. (1986). Hypothesized effect: (+)

Hospital Characteristics		
Location RURAL	*(categorical)* Variable coded as 1 if hospital located in non-MSA; 0 otherwise.	ARF data McKinney, Kaluzny, and Zuckerman (1991). Hypothesized effect: (-)
Teaching status TEACH	*(categorical)* Variable coded as 1 if hospital is a member of the Council of Teaching Hospitals (COTH)	AHA Guide Sloan et al. (1986); Tepelensky et al. (1994). Hypothesized effect: (+)
Size SIZE	*(categorical)* Number of licensed beds	AHA Guide (Schumpeter; P.A. David, 1969; Davies, 1979) Hypothesized effect: (+)
Ownership status NOTPROFT	*(categorical)* Variable coded as 1 if hospital is owned by state, county, city, city-county, hospital district or authority, church or other nongovernmental NFP organization, or the federal government. Coded as 0 if IO hospital	AHA Guide (Rose and Joskow 1990, Kaluzny 1991) Hypothesized effect: (?)

Behavioral Characteristics		
Affiliations AFFILMHS	*(categorical)* Variable coded as 1 if hospital is a member of a multihospital system; 0 otherwise.	Survey McKinney, Kaluzny, and Zuckerman (1991). Hypothesized effect: (+)
Affiliations AFFILGPA	*(categorical)* Variable coded as 1 if hospital is a member of a group purchasing alliance; 0 otherwise.	Survey Hypothesized effect: (+)
Affiliations AFFILIDN	*(categorical)* Variable coded as 1 if hospital is a member of an integrated delivery network; 0 otherwise.	Survey McKinney, Kaluzny, and Zuckerman (1991). Hypothesized effect: (+)
Technological sophistication TECHINDX	*(categorical)* Additive index of technological sophistication, ranging from 0 to 9.	Survey Economists characterize as learning effect (Mansfield); sociologists as 'knowledge' (Rogers) Hypothesized effect: (+)

4.4 Specification of the functional form

The adoption of telemedicine is modeled as a logit in matrix notation,

Equation (2) $\quad L = \ln (P/1\text{-}P) = \alpha + \sum \beta_r X_r$

where L is the log of the odds ratio of adopting telemedicine, and P is the probability that a hospital adopts telemedicine. The X_r are the independent variables—or market, hospital, and behavioral characteristics—that influence the probability of the hospital adopting telemedicine. Thus, the β_r measure the change in the log-odds of adopting telemedicine as the X_r change by a unit. The intercept, α, is the log-odds of adopting telemedicine if the independent variables are all zero

This formulation derives from Griliches' model of hybrid corn diffusion and is a simplified version of subsequent economic diffusion models (Griliches 1957, 1989; Rose and Joskow 1990; Sloan et al.1986; Stoneman 1983; Tepelensky et al. 1994). The primary difference in this formulation, as described and justified previously, is the absence of time as a measure of the dependent variable.

In addition to the precedent in the literature for specifying this type of functional form, the logit has several attractive properties (Gujarati 1988; Maddala 1994).

1. It is mathematically convenient since the probabilities of adoption, P_i , are bounded by 0 and 1.

2. The relationship between the probabilities, P_i , and the independent variables, X_{ir}, is nonlinear, generating a sigmoid or S-shaped curve, which is often assumed to characterize diffusion patterns (Stoneman 1983).

3. Because it uses a maximum likelihood estimation (MLE) technique to calculate the parameter estimates, α_1 and β_{ir}, it is not necessary for the independent variables to be distributed normally in order for the estimates to be consistent.

Thus, the model used in this research project can be written as follows:

Equation (3). $L_i = \ln (Q1ANEW_i/1\text{-}Q1ANEW_i) = \alpha + \beta_1 NEAREST_i + \beta_2 HMOPEN_i + \beta_3 POPULAT + \beta_4 INCOME_i + \beta_5 RURAL_i + \beta_6 TEACH_i + \beta_7 BEDS_i + \beta_8 NOTPROFT_i + \beta_9 AFFILMHS_i + \beta_{10} AFFILGPA_i + \beta_{11} AFFILIDN_i + \beta_{12} TECHINDX_i$

NOTES

1. In fact, the majority of hospitals, 55% in 1988, are classified as private NFP. Moreover, these hospitals accounted for 65% of hospitals beds in 1987 (Hoerger 1991, footnote 1).

2. Using measures of variability in profit, Hoerger (1991) shows that NFP hospitals experience less variability in profit over time, suggesting that these hospitals maximize other variables in addition to profit. Hoerger also notes that profitability varied among NFP hospitals. For example, large NFP hospitals are generally more profitable than small ones, holding geography constant; urban NFP hospitals earn significantly lower profits than rural NFP hospitals; and there was little influence on profits from membership in a multihospital organization, except that government-owned, multihospital members earn significantly lower profits (Hoerger 1991). These results are important in the context of this study because they suggest that ownership and control are important variables to consider when modeling a hospital's economic behavior.

3. This measure becomes particularly problematic in the light of a recent Supreme Court ruling that a hospital's market is more complex than previous definitions acknowledged (*Wall St. Journal*, January 4, 1996, 1).

4. Geopolitical boundaries present similar difficulties to the approach taken by Sloan et al., using MSA- /county-bounded measures: A hospital in another county may be closer for some patients and thus represent competition for the reference hospital.

CHAPTER 5

Research Design and Methods

This chapter details the research design and justifies the survey approach used in this project. It describes data collection, which includes sampling, the survey and follow-up, and the interview process. This chapter also explains the transformation of the survey data into variables used in the diffusion modeling and transformation of the interview data into qualitative narrative. Finally, the chapter identifies and addresses potential validity threats posed by the design of this research project.

5.1 Study design

This project can be characterized as an observational, as opposed to an interventional, study (Stein 1990). The methods of observational research "try to infer causal processes based on observations of concomitancies and sequences as they occur in natural settings, without the advantage of deliberate manipulation and controls to rule out extraneous causal influences" (Cook and Campbell 1979, 295). In such research, the language of experimental or quasi-experimental design is not applicable; thus, there are no pre- or posttest controls.

The unit of analysis for this research is the hospital. This organizational unit of analysis stems from the theoretical perspective that (1) "Structural characteristics of the organization, such as size and complexity," more strongly affect the adoption of innovations in organizational settings than do individual characteristics of people within the organization, and (2) "environmental input from the community and other organizations is a major determinant" of adoption." (Baldridge and Burnham 1975). Using the organization, or hospital, as a unit of analysis is also the convention in economic diffusion models as the organization, rather than the individual, typically invests in the innovation of interest. Since telemedicine technologies represent capital and labor investments of sizable proportions, it is reasonable to pursue a similar approach in this research. Finally, this unit of analysis is also a matter of convenience because it is more tractable than other units, such as doctors' offices or other medical clinics.

Observational research is well suited for understanding telemedicine adoption since changes in behavior relative to some "abrupt and precisely dated" treatment are not the focus of the study (Cook and Campbell 1979). Rather, the focus is first on discovering what types of hospitals will adopt telemedicine, or which units are selecting into a treatment group, before the attempt is made to determine exactly how telemedicine affects the adopters.

This study is analytic, as opposed to purely descriptive, in that it uses theory and empirical evidence to establish causal relationships between selected independent variables and the dependent variable (Stein 1990), which is the probability of adopting telemedicine. It is a cross-sectional, nonlongitudinal study. The time element is not a factor in this research simply because, as described in chapter 4, the observations represent t_0, or an initial point of observation. Therefore, this diffusion study examines the characteristics and predictors of hospitals that would be called "early adopters" in the diffusion literature (Rogers 1983). More important, this study is policy-relevant research. It involves not only the positive, social science techniques of analytic and descriptive modeling, but identifies policy implications and options that derive from this research.

5.2 Survey data collection

This section explains why surveys of hospitals were used to gather information about telemedicine.

5.2.1 Why survey?

The fact that no empirical data currently exist to describe how hospitals are adopting and using telemedicine technologies (Austin and Trimm 1992, Perednia 1995) provides singular justification for conducting primary data collection. Two factors support the decision to use a survey to gather this information. First, the scant information that does exist about telemedicine in the literature consists primarily of reports of individual projects, essentially case studies; thus, the breadth of analysis afforded by a survey is lacking in the literature. Second, survey methodology is the appropriate technique to apply to identify systematic patterns (Yin 1984) of technology adoption across different hospital environments, which include variations in size, ownership status, membership in multihospital systems, and geographic location. Moreover, the survey was supplemented by numerous telephone and in-person interviews with hospital administrators and telemedicine project managers. Supplemental interviews helped to compensate for the depth of information the survey could not capture.

5.2.2 Sampling

There are 152 hospitals in North Carolina, 88 in South Carolina, and 166 in Georgia. To avoid comparing dissimilar units of analysis, only hospitals that the 1994 American Hospital Association *Guide to Hospitals in the U.S.* classifies as *general* hospitals were investigated. These are hospitals whose

"primary function . . . is to provide patient services, diagnostic and therapeutic, for a variety of medical conditions. A general hospital shall provide: diagnostic x-ray services with facilities and staff for a variety of procedures, clinical laboratory service with facilities and staff for a variety of procedures and with anatomical pathology services . . ., and operating room service with facilities and staff (AHA *Guide*, 1992,A5).

This distinction eliminates *special* hospitals, whose "primary function . . . is to provide diagnostic and treatment services for patients who have specified medical conditions, both surgical and nonsurgical" (AHA *Guide*, 1992, A5). For example, special hospitals would include children's hospitals, rehabilitation hospitals, long-term care hospitals, and osteopathic hospitals. Limiting the investigation to general hospitals also eliminates *psychiatric* hospitals, whose "primary function . . . is to provide diagnostic and treatment services for patients who have psychiatric-related illnesses" (AHA *Guide*, 1992,A5). These would include state-run and private psychiatric hospitals, as well as hospitals that specialize in substance abuse.

In North Carolina, there are 123 general hospitals. South Carolina has 69 general hospitals, and Georgia has 157. These total to 349 general hospitals in the sample, a number that allows for a manageable census and eliminates stratification issues.

5.2.3 Survey logistics

The survey was mailed directly to the chief administrator of each hospital. The chief administrator was expected either to complete the survey personally or to forward the survey to the appropriate individual(s). This approach involved a degree of risk of increasing the nonresponse rate if the surveys were passed among more than one respondent in a hospital. Unfortunately, this risk could not be avoided: Due to the complexity and breadth of the survey, along with the diversity of hospitals' personnel duties, identifying a more appropriate individual a priori was impossible. Furthermore, in the majority of cases, the administrator was the most appropriate respondent.

To minimize the potential for nonresponse, it was critical that the administrators felt interested in the subject and/or obligated to reply. To that end, I enlisted the help and influence of the hospital associations of each state. Nearly all hospitals belong to associations; these organizations lobby on behalf of the hospitals. Each state hospital association wrote a letter of support for the study, urging their members to participate. This letter was included in the survey mailing (Appendix D).

5.2.4   Survey development

During November and December 1994, the survey was developed. The pilot survey was based on a framework devised from the research proposal and its economic cost model. The items of interest included hospitals' output levels (for example, number of patients discharged per year) and prices of inputs (including labor, medical and pharmaceutical supplies). Also included were hospitals' investments in telemedicine and administrative information technologies.

This framework was the basis of interviews with over 14 individuals (Appendix A), including hospital administrators, telemedicine coordinators, hospital association executives, and other researchers in telemedicine. The interviews were structured around the pilot survey and probed appropriate terminology, internal accounting practices, and the relevancy of items on the questionnaire.

The final survey was developed using the comments from these interviews, a preliminary review of the literature on the diffusion of medical technologies, and Dillman's (1978) chapters on "Writing Questions," and "Constructing Mail Questionnaires." The survey was sent to 349 general hospitals in North Carolina, South Carolina, and Georgia. While the primary objective of the questionnaire was to obtain data for the economic cost model, questions relevant to the diffusion of telemedicine were included for two reasons. First, a diffusion framework was necessary to test for endogeneity in the proposed cost model. In other words, it was necessary to obtain information about characteristics of the hospital that might be associated with the adoption of telemedicine; these same characteristics might also be associated with lower operating costs independent of investments in telemedicine. Second, it was recognized at the outset of this project that the necessary financial data to construct the cost model would be difficult to obtain. In the event that the cost-modeling data were incomplete, the questionnaire included several items that would allow for the development of a diffusion model. Therefore, this survey aimed to obtain the necessary data to construct an economic cost model and the diffusion model, as well as to gather information about administrators' perceived barriers to adoption and the medical applications for which hospitals are currently using telemedicine.

5.2.5   Survey mailing

Following Dillman's (1978) guidelines, the surveys were mailed to hospital administrators. Each mailing included a personalized cover letter that explained the importance and interest of this study and assured the confidentiality of answers. To provide every opportunity for response, the cover letter and survey specified a fax number for returning the survey if the respondent would prefer this option to using the mail. The first mailing included two enclosures: (1) a 1-page description of the study, its sponsors, and its policy-relevance and (2) a letter of support from the appropriate state's hospital association. A preprinted envelope with prepaid return postage was enclosed with these materials and was mailed on March 25, 1995.

Again, according to Dillman's guidelines (1978), a postcard reminder was sent after the initial mailing. Because the survey was complex and was possibly being circulated to more than one individual, the reminder was sent 2 weeks after the initial mailing (rather than Dillman's prescribed 1 week). Hospitals that had not already answered earlier mailings were sent two subsequent rounds of repeat survey mailings, followed at 2 weeks with postcard reminders. Reminders were mailed, respectively, at 6 and 8 weeks and 12 and 14 weeks after the initial mailing. Each round of mailings included a 1-page description of the study, a personalized cover letter, and a return postage-paid envelope. Telephone follow-ups were implemented after the second and third rounds of mailings. These calls encouraged the administrators of the nonresponding hospitals to complete and return the questionnaire. The calls also provided an opportunity, when possible, to obtain the survey data and other contextual information over the telephone.

5.3 Qualitative data

This research also involved qualitative data collection in the form of interviews with key informants. Between March 1995 and March 1996, over 40 interviews took place either over the telephone or in-person. Three types of interviews were conducted. The first type of interview was a telephone interview, structured around the survey. The primary objective of this type of interview was to obtain key items of interest from the survey. In many cases, these interviews supplied the forum to elicit more detailed information about the plans and attitudes of administrators regarding telemedicine.

The second type of interview supplemented the survey data. Survey respondents and key informants were identified and subsequently interviewed over the telephone. At the outset of the telephone call, the interviewer indicated that these conversations would last less than 5 minutes. Stating the time limit was an important strategy because administrative assistants invariably screened the administrators' calls. Stating the purpose and brevity of the call made contacting administrators easie. The purpose of these calls was to establish the linkages among telemedicine projects in the sample and to determine how hospitals plan to finance their telemedicine projects in the future.

The third type of interviews was conducted both over the telephone and in-person. These sessions focused on managed care issues and again involved key informants. These informants were identified according to their familiarity with more evolved managed care markets. Seeking informants from both the region of study in the survey and from other regions allowed potential variation in strategies, attitudes, and relationships between telemedicine and managed care to be captured. These interviews were loosely structured around the concepts in the diffusion model, but were purposefully open ended to explore whether a relationship existed between telemedicine and managed and to probe the nature of this relationship.

5.4 Variable construction

The construction of the variables included in the diffusion model was relatively straightforward. Many variables were simply direct measures of the concept of interest. This section will identify each of the major concepts included in the model and will explain the variables measuring these concepts.

5.4.1 The dependent variable

Adoption of telemedicine is the categorical dependent variable, which was supplied by Question 1.a. of the survey. This variable was coded as "1" if the responding hospital had adopted telemedicine and "0" if it had not.

5.4.2 Market characteristics

Competition from other hospitals in a given hospital's local market is measured as the distance to the next nearest hospital to the hospital being observed. This variable was constructed using the Area Resource Files

(ARF) to identify hospital zip codes as a geographic reference point. The distance between each hospital and all the other hospitals in the data set was then calculated; from this, the minimum distance was identified and assigned as the NEAREST variable. The natural log of this variable was calculated and the transformed variable was used in calculations in order to compress the scale and reduce the influence of very small and very large values.

The other measure of market competitiveness, the percentage of the population in the metropolitan statistical area (MSA) or county enrolled in a health maintenance organization (HMO), was also constructed from the ARF data. The ARF data supplied the number of individuals enrolled in an HMO enrollment per county. This figure was simply summed for MSAs, divided by the county or MSA population, and multiplied by 100 to convert decimals to percentages. Similarly, the demand characteristics of the market were taken directly from the ARF data, where population and per capita income of the counties are reported or summed from the county-level data for MSAs. POPULAT, the variable representing population, was calculated by first scaling the population of the county or MSA by 1000 and then taking the natural log of this figure to compress the scale and diminish the leverage of the very large MSAs on the analysis. INCOME, the variable representing county or MSA incomes, was simply the per capita income of the county (in $100s), or the weighted average of the per capita incomes of the counties (in $100s) that constitute an MSA. For the purposes of analysis, this variable was scaled by a factor of 100 in the regression analysis to improve interpretation of the odds coefficients and odds ratios.[1]

5.4.3   Hospital characteristics

Again, these five variables were very simply constructed. The variable that accounts for hospital location is categorical: RURAL was simply coded as "1" if the hospital is not located in an MSA and "0" if it is located in an MSA. Teaching status is represented by a categorical variable, TEACH, which was coded as "1" if the hospital is a member of the Council of Teaching Hospitals and coded as "0" if otherwise. The size variable, BEDS, is simply a continuous variable, using the number of licensed beds to represent the size of the hospital. As with NEAREST and

POPULAT, this variable was logged to compress the scale. Ownership status is represented as a dummy variable, NOTPROFT, if the hospital is not-for-profit and coded as "0" if otherwise. These categories were aggregated from ownership data from the American Hospital Association.

5.4.4 Behavioral characteristics

Hospitals were categorized by affiliation according to the survey data. Dummy variables represent membership in multihospital systems (AFFILMHS), group purchasing alliances (AFFILGPA), and integrated delivery networks (AFFILIDN).

Technological sophistication is measured as an additive index, which is a continuous variable ranging between 0 and 9. The technologies included in this index are representative of two types of hospital information systems: inventory management and medical records. Within each category, technologies were included that exemplify increasing degrees of technological sophistication. Thus, the inventory management technologies included in the index are as follows: (1) computerized inventory management, (2) computerized accounts payable, (3) internally networked inventory management, (4) off-site inventory areas electronically linked to main inventory management system (e.g., with wide-area-networks (WAN), leased telephone lines, microwave transmissions, or modems), (5) stockless or just-in-time (JIT) inventory management, and (6) accounts payable managed by electronic data interexchange (EDI) for at least some accounts. These technologies account for both the purchasing and the payment aspects of inventory management. They also represent a parallel step-wise progression in technological sophistication. For example, it is impossible to have internally networked inventory management without first having computerized inventory management. Similarly, stockless or JIT inventory management relies on networked computers; EDI depends on first having computerized accounts payable. The medical records technologies included in the index were (1) computerized admissions, discharge, and transfer (ADT) records management, (2) partially computerized medical records management, and (3) medical records available electronically to remote affiliated clinical sites. Again, these technologies represent a step-wise progression in technological sophistication.

TECHINDX was constructed in a stepwise fashion. First, each of nine types of information technologies was coded as "1" if the hospital had adopted the technology at the time of the survey or planned to adopt in 1995; otherwise, the technology was coded as "0." Second, the index was created by summing these nine categories. Hospitals with the least sophisticated technologies and the fewest technologies score lower than those with more sophisticated or more technologies. For example, a hospital that has internally networked inventory systems, but no medical records technologies would score similarly to a hospital with less sophisticated inventory management, but with some medical records technologies. The TECHINDX variable, therefore, accounts for the presence of multiple types of information systems and various levels of sophistication within each type of information system.

This approach is consistent with the technique used by Kimberly and Evanisko (1981), whereby they defined adoption of a class of technologies to be "the sum of the respective number of innovations reported by the hospital administrator." This type of summated index is criticized on the basis that the index ignores variations within a particular innovation that is a component of the index, and thus ignores the potential influence of this variability on adoption decisions. This caution is warranted, but the use and construction of the TECHINDX in this research limit the definitions of the constituent categories of technologies in order to minimize the danger of variability.

5.5 Validity threats

While every attempt was made to design this study as rigorously as possible, potential threats to the validity of the conclusions drawn from this research warrant discussion.

5.5.1 Construct validity

Construct validity refers to the fit between the measurement of a concept and the theoretical construct the measurement is designed to represent (Cook and Campbell 1979). Three potential threats to construct validity are present in this research. The first is the internal validity of the constructs themselves: Key elements of this research relied on information reported by individual hospital administrators. Therefore, the strength of the conclusions depends on the accuracy of their responses. The hospital administrator or survey respondent may not accurately report whether a hospital has adopted telemedicine or what types of telemedicine projects are active. As explained in chapter 2, due to the early stage of telemedicine evolution, in many hospitals, it is possible that there is "no one . . . who knows about all the telemedicine activities."[2] Moreover, the possibility exists that hospitals would inaccurately report adoption or plans to adopt telemedicine in 1995 and falsely qualify as an adopter for this study. Inaccurate reporting could be attributed either to the desire to be perceived as technologically sophisticated or to unforeseen delays in project implementation. The latter possibility is less threatening to the study than the former. Nonetheless, such difficulties are not uncharacteristic of survey research. The only alternative design that would eliminate such dangers would be a site visit to verify the telemedicine projects of each responding hospital. For obvious reasons, such an approach would be impossible.

The second type of potential threat to construct validity refers to potential mismeasurement of theoretical concepts. As explained in chapters 3 and 4, the majority of the constructs, or variables included in the model, are clearly defined by theory and have been used extensively in the literature. While problems may exist, these constructs are the best available and allow for comparison between studies. The one new construct introduced into this research is the index TECHINDX, measuring technological sophistication. The index could be problematic because it assumes an additive relationship between the technologies that are components of the index and the idea of technological sophistication. Thus, a hospital with a TECHINDX score of 8 is assumed to be twice as technologically sophisticated as a hospital with a score of 4.

Nonetheless, the advantages of the TECHINDX measure outweigh the disadvantages for two important reasons. The first reason in that the index uses primary data, not available elsewhere. While other measures of the sophistication of medical technologies within a hospital are available, this index is the only source of information about information systems. Thus, the precision of this index in measuring administrative technological sophistication is superior to other potential proxies for technological sophistication. The second reason is that the method by which this variable was constructed attempted to take advantage of the additive properties of an index, including technologies that are progressively more sophisticated. This reason, combined with a lack of evidence to the contrary, make the implicit assumption of additivity a necessity and reasonable.

The third way that construct validity threat is used in this research is to connote the possibility that the information gathered from key informants may suffer from biases related to the biases of these individuals. As Lofland and Lofland (1984, 42) explain, "The understanding of these helpers may, of course, be erroneous or misleading, and the wise investigator is never too gullible." In order to minimize the potential threat that the informants' biases may pose to the conclusions, multiple sources were contacted for these interviews.

5.5.2 External validity

External validity, or the ability to generalize to a larger population from the results of this research, is threatened to the extent that hospitals in the three states examined differ from hospitals in other regions of the United States. Three factors may limit generalizability. First, due to word of mouth, or regionally developed social networks, hospitals in the three states may have greater or lesser knowledge about telemedicine than hospitals in other regions. Second, the geography and demography of the three states are somewhat unique in the United States. In contrast to regions in the western United States, distances between hospitals in these three states are relatively short, and populations are relatively more evenly dispersed. In contrast to the Northeastern corridor or the Western and Plains states, the populations of this region are relatively evenly dispersed between rural and urban areas. Since telemedicine is an inherently distance-sensitive technology, these regional differences may limit generalizability. Finally, the health care markets of these three states are each relatively less developed in terms of managed care than other regions of the United States (Curran and O'Connor 1995; *Hospitals & Health Networks* 1995; Kripke Byers and Levi-Baumgarten 1995). To the extent that managed care influences the diffusion of telemedicine technologies, this factor could limit the generalizability of the study. Because the region of study shares many population, health care market, and demographic similarities with enough other regions of the United States, this research, despite its limitations, is useful outside the region.

NOTES

1. POPULAT and INCOME are scaled for two reasons: (1) to improve the interpretation of the coefficients; for example, odds ratios make more sense and are more policy- relevant when the margin of change refers to $100 in per capita income, rather than per $1 and (2) POPULAT is logged, in addition to scaling by 1,000, to compress the scale and reduce the leverage of the larger cities in the analysis.

2. Personal communication, 11/8-12/95. Dr. Henry Hsiao, Professor of Biomedical Engineering, UNC-CH.

CHAPTER 6

Characteristics of the Survey Population and Descriptive Statistics

This chapter characterizes the context of this research project. Information about the distribution of population, hospitals and hospital beds is provided, along with a comparison of these features among the three states. The chapter also explains the relevant telecommunications and telemedicine policies of each state. In addition, this chapter describes the study population in terms of the survey questions and responses. It provides background information obtained from the survey and from qualitative research, which serves as a backdrop for the data and analyses of the diffusion modeling. Finally, the chapter supplies summary statistics for the variables included in the diffusion model and reports the results of bivariate analyses of the relationships between the independent variables of the diffusion model and the dependent variable, adoption of telemedicine.

6.1 Characteristics of the research context

This section describes North Carolina, South Carolina, and Georgia in terms of the distribution of population and hospitals. This region was chosen as the context for this research for two reasons: (1) Since this research was conducted from Chapel Hill, North Carolina, the choice of three contiguous southeastern states was obvious and convenient. (2) Moreover, this region includes two states with policies designed to encourage the development and adoption of telemedicine and telecommunications applications. North Carolina has pursued one of the most aggressive telecommunications policies in the United States; the result is a very sophisticated, statewide telecommunications infrastructure. Georgia boasts the most extensive state-sponsored distance learning and telemedicine network. These two states provide a fertile environment for telemedicine. Consequently, examining the diffusion of telemedicine in these states and in South Carolina, where state policies have not been as aggressive, was interesting. This chapter makes a case for considering the three states as a homogeneous region, based on these characteristics. Finally, the chapter compares and contrasts the policies of each state regarding telemedicine and the supporting telecommunications infrastructure.

6.1.1 Population

Table 6-1 illustrates the populations and their geographic distributions for North Carolina, South Carolina, and Georgia.

Table 6-1. Population Characteristics and Distribution of Study States

	North Carolina	South Carolina	Georgia	South Atlantic	U.S.
Population (1,000s) in 1994	7,070	3,664	7,055	46,398	260,341
1994 U.S. population rank	10	25	11	NA	NA
1994 population density (population/ square mile)	145.1	121.7	121.8	174.3	73.6
Percentage of population living in MSAs 1992	66.3	69.8	67.7	78.9	79.7
Percentage of pop. living outside MSAs in 1992	33.7	30.2	32.3	21.1	20.3

Source: Statistical Abstract of the U.S. 1995

North Carolina and Georgia are comparable in terms of population, whereas South Carolina has just over one half the population of these states. In each of the three states, roughly one third of the population lives in nonmetropolitan, or rural, areas. This contrasts to the South Atlantic region[1] as a whole, where only 21% of the population lives in nonmetropolitan areas. The population densities, or persons per square mile, are also relatively comparable in the three states, with North Carolina being slightly more densely settled than Georgia and South Carolina. The three states are substantially less densely populated than the region as a whole. The population densities, however, do not paint a very clear picture of the geographic distribution of the states' populations.

Tables 6-2 through 6-4 provide more detailed information, describing the population distributions among the urban centers of the three states.

In North Carolina, the urban population is distributed among 12 metropolitan statistical areas (MSAs). The large number of MSAs shows a relatively evenly distributed population (Table 6-2 and Figure 6-1).

Table 6-2. MSAs in North Carolina

Metropolitan Area	1992 Population
Goldsboro	107,712
Greenville	112,426
Wilmington	127,808
Rocky Mount	136,734
Jacksonville	144,531
Norfolk-Virginia Beach-Newport News[2] (Currituck County, NC)	147,630
Asheville	197,463
Fayetteville	277,322
Hickory-Morganton	299,218
Raleigh-Durham-Chapel Hill	909,232
Greensboro-Winston-Salem-High Point	1,078,377
Charlotte-Gastonia-Rock Hill, NC-SC	1,212,393

Source: Area Resource Files 1995.

Figure 6-1 North Carolina Metropolitan Statistical Areas

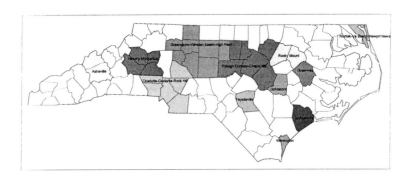

In South Carolina, the Charlotte-Gastonia, NC-Rock Hill, SC MSA has the largest population, but much of this population lives on the North Carolina side of the border.

Table 6-3. MSAs in South Carolina

Metropolitan Area	1992 Population
Sumter	105,356
Florence	118,595
Myrtle Beach	152,321
Augusta, GA-Aiken, SC	422,660
Columbia	471,837
Charleston-North Charleston	528,587
Greenville-Spartanburg-Anderson	852,962
Charlotte-Gastonia, NC-Rock Hill, SC	1,212,393

Source: Area Resource Files 1995.

Figure 6-2   South Carolina Metropolitan Statistical Areas

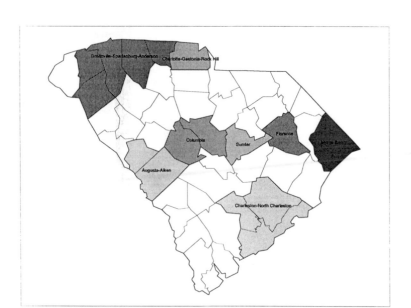

In Georgia, the population is more concentrated than in North or South Carolina. Nearly one half of Georgia's population lives in the Atlanta MSA. The rest of Georgia's population, however, is distributed relatively evenly between the other seven much smaller MSAs and the rural areas.

Table 6-4. MSAs in Georgia

Metropolitan Area	1992 Population
Albany	115,232
Chatenooga, TN	116,914
Athens	128,970
Columbus	220,939
Savannah	267,360
Macon	298,625
Agusta, GA-Aiken, SC	422,660
Atlanta	3,142,857

Figure 6-3 Georgia Metropolitan Statistical Areas

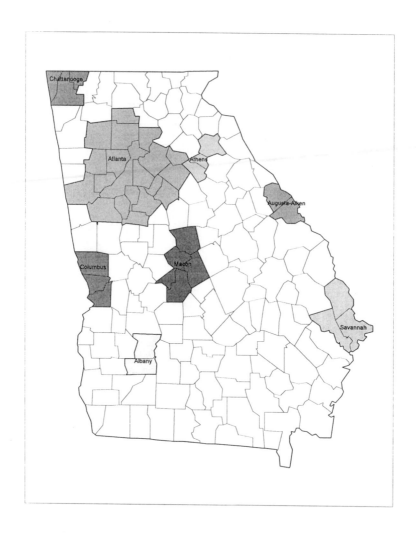

6.1.2 Hospital characteristics

In addition to understanding the distribution of the population in the study area, it is also important to gain perspective on the accessibility of hospital care in the region; i.e., does the distribution of the population match the distribution of hospitals? This information is relevant to research on telemedicine because it provides some indication of the distance rural residents typically travel to receive hospital care. Table 6-5 describes the distribution of hospitals and hospital beds in the three study states.

Table 6-5. Basic Hospital Statistics of Study States

	North Carolina	South Carolina	Georgia	South Atlantic	U.S.
Number of general hospitals	123	69	157	790	5,261
Number of general hospitals in MSAs	57 (46%)	50 (72%)	64 (41%)	Not Available	Not Available
Beds in general hospitals	22,430	10,770	24,929	159,100	916,200
Beds in MSAs	15,604 (70%)	8,213 (76%)	17,141 (69%)	Not Available	Not Available

Sources: 1994 AHA *Guide*, Statistical Abstract of the U.S.

The information presented in Table 6-5 indicates that less than one half of the hospitals in North Carolina and Georgia are located in urban areas, whereas 72% of South Carolina's hospitals are in urban areas. Thus, rural residents of North Carolina and Georgia seem to have greater access to hospital care than do their neighbors in South Carolina. Comparing the location of hospital beds, however, paints a more subtle picture. In each of the three states, approximately 70% of all hospital beds are located in urban areas; slightly under 70% of the population of these states live in urban areas. North Carolina and Georgia have many very small hospitals in their rural areas, while South Carolina has proportionally fewer but larger hospitals located in its nonmetropolitan regions. As with the statistics describing the states' populations, the hospital statistics reveal important similarities among the states, which warrant treating the three states as a relatively homogeneous region (Figure 6-4).

Figure 6-4 Distribution of Hospitals in the Study Region

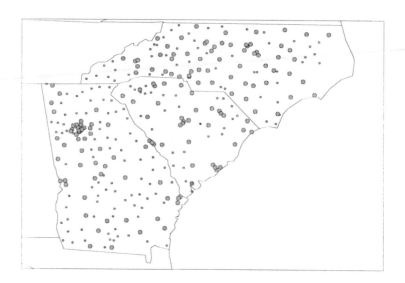

6.1.3 Telecommunications and telemedicine policies

North Carolina. Of the three states studied, North Carolina has implemented the most aggressive initiative, the North Carolina Integrated Information Network (NCIIN), to develop a telecommunications network (Office of the State Controller 1996). With an announcement of a $4.4 million investment, the state introduced the NCIIN, which was intended to "improve education and health care for residents of the state's poorer counties; and bring sophisticated industries with higher-paying jobs to North Carolina" (*Raleigh News & Observer*, May 11, 93). While the three goals of the NCIIN focus on economic development, telemedicine is an explicit component of the state's vision for applications of the NCIIN. In 1994, as part of the NCIIN initiative, the Office of the Governor created a nonprofit public-private partnership, the North Carolina Health Care Information and Communications Alliance (NCHCICA), designed to support the development of health care applications on the NCIIN (Lipson and Henderson 1995). In addition, the state played a central role in the application for, and implementation of, a federal grant project (funded by the Department of Commerce's National Telecommunications and Information Administration, or NTIA), which was awarded to the state's four academic medical centers. The NTIA grant supports linkages between rural hospitals and the emergency departments of the Duke University Medical Center, the University of North Carolina Hospitals, Bowman-Gray School of Medicine, and East Carolina University. Although telemedicine is not the primary focus of state policy, the state of North Carolina provides considerable support for telemedicine as part of its broader initiative to develop the NCIIN and establish viable applications for the NCIIN.

South Carolina. The state government of South Carolina has little involvement with telemedicine activities. Nor does the state have a specific policy for promoting the development of a sophisticated telecommunications network. In contrast to many states, however, South Carolina's relatively liberal telecommunications policy poses few regulatory or legal barriers to cooperation between the state's telecommunications providers. As a result, consortia of independent telephone companies have evolved, deploying fiber-optic technologies across the state much more quickly than would have been possible in the absence of this cooperation (Office of Technology Assessment 1991). To the extent that such advanced communications technologies are essential to the development of telemedicine, South Carolina provides a hospitable, if not explicitly proactive, policy backdrop for the growth of these technologies.

Georgia. The state of Georgia touts its telemedicine system, the Georgia Statewide Academic and Medical System (GSAMS), as "the largest and most comprehensive distance learning and health care network in the world" (GSAMS 1996). With the passage of the Distance Learning and Telemedicine Act of 1992 (SB 144), Georgia launched the largest state-sponsored telemedicine initiative in the United States. By the provisions of this legislation, $50 million of excess earnings of the telephone company were allocated to a fund to finance telecommunications projects in medicine and education, rather than refunded directly to consumers. Of these funds, $8 million was directly allocated to telemedicine projects (Anderson and Sanders 1993). This legislation also established a governing board for the GSAMS, which sets policies, reviews applications, and awards funding for the network (Lipson and Henderson 1995). By October of 1995, 57 telemedicine sites were operational (GSAMS 1996), giving Georgia the most telemedicine sites of any state in the United States. This network crisscrosses the state, reaching from the academic medical centers to remote and rural hospitals across the state. The 1996 Olympic Games gave even further impetus for telemedicine development, providing justification to link hospitals proximate to the sailing and rowing venues, which were far from Atlanta, to the Medical College of Georgia in Augusta and Emory University in Atlanta[3].

More important, at the time of this study, Georgia was also the only state for which the Health Care Financing Administration (HCFA) had granted limited Medicare reimbursement for telemedicine consultations (Lipson and Henderson 1995). In addition, Georgia's Medicaid program and Blue Cross/Blue Shield reimburse for telemedical consultations—at the time of this research, Georgia was the only state in which physicians were reimbursed for telemedical consultations by Medicare, Medicaid, or other third-party payers. As will be explained further, hospital administrators identified the lack of reimbursement as an important barrier to the development of telemedicine; with insurers reimbursing for telemedicine consults, this barrier was not a factor in Georgia. Georgia's aggressive programs to finance and facilitate the development of telemedicine projects, along with a favorable insurance environment, unquestionably promoted the extensive telemedicine network that exists in the state.

6.2 Background information

This section describes the survey responses and synthesizes information gathered from the survey with information obtained in interviews with hospital administrators, physicians, and telemedicine coordinators. The individuals interviewed for this project were extraordinarily candid in their comments. For this reason, quotations are not attributed to individuals. Rather, a list of interview participants is provided in the appendix. The information presented in this section provides a backdrop for the data and analysis from the diffusion modeling.

6.2.1 Response and adoption rates

Table 6-6 summarizes statistics about the population, the respondents, and telemedicine adopters.

Table 6-6. Population, Response, Adoption, and Rural Location

Group	Total N	Rural (Non-MSA)	Urban (MSA)	χ^2 (prob) {Fisher's Exact Test: 2-Tail}
Population	349	186 (53%)	163 (47%)	N/A
Respondents	166 (48% of pop.)	100 (60% of respond-ents)	66 (40% of respond-ents)	$\chi^2 = 6.13$ (P= 0.013) {0.014}
Telemedicine Adopters	66 (40% of respond-ents)	32 (48% of adopters)	34 (52% of adopters)	$\chi^2 = 6.32$ (P= 0.012) {0.015}

The 349 hospitals in the study population were approximately evenly divided between rural (53%) and urban (47%) locations, with slightly more rural hospitals in the region. A total of 166 (48%) of the hospitals in the population responded to the survey. Proportionally more rural hospitals responded to the survey than are represented in the population. This bias was statistically significant, as indicated by the low probability[4] (0.013) of a chi-square score of 6.13. This bias created an imperative to weight the model to compensate for the fact that the respondents did not accurately represent the population for this characteristic. Of the respondents, 66 (40%) reported adopting telemedicine. Of the telemedicine adopters, 32 (48%) were rural hospitals and 34 (52%) were urban hospitals. Given that urban hospitals were statistically underrepresented among respondents, they were overrepresented among telemedicine adopters. This urban bias in telemedicine adoption was statistically significant ($\chi^2 = 6.32$; p = 0.012).

6.2.2 Hospital strategy and the role of telemedicine

Table 6-7 describes the responses of telemedicine adopters to questions about the role of telemedicine in their hospital's strategic, or competitive, plans. These questions asked the hospitals to rank on a Likert scale, ranging from 1 (not at all important) to 5 (very important), how important to their competitive strategies they considered the adoption of telemedicine to be.

Table 6-7. Strategic Importance of Telemedicine

Importance of Telemedicine	Highly Important
Providing quality health care in the local market	72%
Technological leadership in the local market	69%
Managed care strategy	63%
Price competitiveness in the local market	25%

To be considered highly important, telemedicine had to be ranked by the hospitals as a 4 or 5 on the Likert-scaled questions. Thus, 38 hospitals, or 63%of adopters, reported that adoption of telemedicine was highly important to their managed care strategy. Of the 51 (81%) adopters who stated that they faced competition in their local market, 13 (25%) ranked the adoption of telemedicine as highly important to their price competitiveness in the local market; 35 (69%) stated that the adoption of telemedicine was highly important to the hospital's role as a technological leader in the local market; and 37 (72%) maintained that telemedicine adoption was highly important to providing quality health care in the local market.

These results were interesting because they reflected the self-reported importance of telemedicine adoption to various competitive strategies. As such, it is important to keep in mind that the range of socially appropriate responses may have been narrower than the actual range of the Likert scale. For example, administrators would be unlikely to answer that telemedicine was less than highly important to delivering quality health care in the local market. Therefore, caution in interpreting these results is warranted. Nonetheless, the responses reflected strategic perspectives about telemedicine that had not yet been explored. The fact that 69% of the adopters in competitive markets indicated that telemedicine adoption was highly important to their role as technological leaders in the local market place demonstrated an important marketing function that telemedicine may perform. Similarly, few hospitals (25%) in this group indicated that telemedicine was highly important to their price competitiveness in the local market. This result suggested the possibility that most administrators did not expect telemedicine to reduce costs sufficiently to warrant a corresponding price reduction. Another possibility is that administrators had not thoroughly calculated the potential price and cost impacts of telemedicine. Either way, these results showed that the financial impact of telemedicine was overshadowed by the potential marketing effect.

Subsequent to the survey, interviews with hospital administrators helped to further elucidate the reasons administrators identified for adopting telemedicine. Four reasons were prominent among the administrators interviewed. The most commonly cited reason was marketing, followed by improving care in remote locations, extending medical education, and reducing the cost of care. Without prompting from the interviewer, administrators never independently identified a role of telemedicine in a managed care strategy. Their thoughts about this subject were nonetheless very interesting.

Marketing. When questioned as to why their hospitals adopted telemedicine, administrators invariably related telemedicine to some aspect of marketing. One chief financial officer summed up the hospital's decision to adopt telemedicine in one word: "Positioning." Another administrator of a rural hospital said that telemedicine adoption was driven by patients' requests: "Patients expect high-tech assistance. It makes them feel special. The physicians feel that it's a gimmick." He went on to explain that telemedicine did not change how physicians at his hospital practice medicine, rather it made his hospital competitive because patients demanded state-of-the-art technologies. In the words of another administrator, "We see everybody else turning to telemedicine, and we know we need to keep up."

One hospital administrator likened telemedicine to clinical consultation services, where physicians in remote areas dial a toll-free number to receive consultations from a tertiary care center. The tertiary care center offers this service in an effort to establish relationships and referral patterns between the physicians and the hospital. This administrator saw telemedicine as an extension of a consultation service.

Quality of care. After marketing, the ability to improve access to health care in rural areas was the next most frequently specified reason for adopting telemedicine. One administrator of a tertiary care hospital indicated that the impetus to adopt telemedicine came from the rural hospitals affiliated with this larger hospital. The rural hospitals seemed convinced that telemedicine could bring higher quality care to their communities. This administrator characterized the arrangement as win-win: the rural areas received improved care, and the urban hospital gained or solidified referral patterns. The telemedicine director at another tertiary care center echoed this story. Rural hospitals affiliated with the tertiary care center were seeking assistance at a time when the larger hospital was examining its strategic planning for the next 5 years; telemedicine fit the objectives of all parties involved.

Other rural hospitals indicated that they had adopted teleradiology out of necessity: Few or no radiologists practiced in their communities. In order to gain access to radiologic services, they adopted telemedicine. In several cases, radiologists in other communities shared the cost of the system. Radiology was the only specialty mentioned in the context of the medical necessity of adopting telemedicine.

Medical Education. Among those interviewed, one hospital administrator stated that medical education was of primary importance in his hospital's adoption of telemedicine. Interactive video connections with a medical school over 100 miles away allowed this rural hospital with only 42 beds to offer a residency program for rural primary care physicians. For a hospital this size to run a residency program is unprecedented.

Several administrators explained that, while not the primary reason, medical education served as a supporting rationale for adopting telemedicine. There are two ways that telemedicine can play this role. The most obvious is the analogy between telemedicine and distance learning. Hospitals can subscribe to, or offer, continuing medical education using teleconferencing technologies. One physician, who had used telemedicine, described a more subtle form of medical education. In this form, the remote physician learns from the specialist in the urban center when a consultation occurs; the rural doctor, when next encountering a similar case, will better know how to treat it before engaging in a telemedical consultation. One administrator explained how he expected this transfer of skills to also reduce the cost of care, as physicians share "best practice" guidelines using telemedicine.

Managed care. Few hospitals among those surveyed and interviewed identified an explicit strategic role for telemedicine in their long-range plans to adapt to managed care. One hospital indicated plans to supply telemedicine consultations on a contract basis. For a negotiated flat rate, the hospital would provide clinical consultations in a variety of specialties to other hospitals or physicians' practices. In essence, this hospital planned to establish its own capitated pricing for telemedicine. Another administrator explained that under managed care, hospitals face an incentive to avoid bringing patients into the hospital, where care is expensive. In his words, "Under managed care, you want to keep 'em down on the farm, where it's cheaper." Therefore, telemedicine, by allowing patients to remain in their communities, could be an important component of a managed care strategy. This same administrator also stressed that this technology could help him to be more competitive in a managed care environment because patients who stay in their own communities would expend less travel time to receive care and thus experience greater satisfaction. Other hospital administrators painted scenarios where, under a capitated pricing regime, they could foresee using telemedicine to reduce costs in outlying affiliated medical centers or in clinics by substituting telemedicine for a reduced staff. For a hospital or clinic that now employs a general practitioner or internist and supplements this care with specialty consultations using telemedicine, all or some of the physician's time could be replaced by a midlevel practitioner supplemented with telemedicine.

The majority of administrators interviewed indicated no explicit strategy for using telemedicine to gain advantage in a managed care environment. As one administrator in North Carolina explained,

"In our region, no one is further than 45 miles from a primary care provider. The personal contact is too important to people: they will drive for an hour to see a physician. Where telemedicine comes in, is for specialty visits. But I can't imagine substituting the technology for a professional for primary care visits."

This perspective illustrates two important points. First, this administrator recognizes the potential for reducing costs by substituting telemedicine for physicians in a capitated pricing environment. Second, he dismisses this strategy in markets like that of central North Carolina, where distances to the nearest primary care provider are relatively small. He believes that people value personal contact enough that his hospital would lose patients to the competition if his hospital used telemedicine as a substitute for a primary care physician. As he continued to think aloud about this issue, his comments echoed those of other administrators. In a capitated pricing environment, several administrators reasoned that using telemedicine to access specialty consults would be less expensive than transporting patients to a tertiary care center. Thus, telemedicine could allow smaller hospitals to improve their competitiveness by increasing the mix of services they could offer and by reducing their cost of providing these services. Among this group of administrators, however, such a strategy was not an explicit component of their reasons for adopting telemedicine.

For the most part, the interviews confirmed the survey results as to why hospitals were adopting telemedicine. Moreover, price competitiveness was never brought up by administrators. When asked directly about this issue, most paused to think about it, but responded that it was too early to tell how costs and prices would be determined for telemedicine-related activities.

6.2.3 Financing telemedicine

Question 2 on the survey asked hospitals to rank the sources of capital for telemedicine projects in order of the largest dollar amounts. Table 6-8 summarizes these results.

Table 6-8. Sources of Capital for Telemedicine Projects

Most Important Source	Frequency
1. Operating revenues	24 (38%)
2. Federal grants	10 (16%)
3. Other sources	6 (9.5%)
4. State grants	5 (8%)
5. Foundation grants	4 (6.3%)
6. Other hospital sources	1 (1.6%)
7. Affiliated hospitals	1 (1.5%)

The category most often indicated as the primary source of telemedicine funds was operating revenues; 38% of telemedicine adopters ranked this category highest. In this sample, federal grants accounted for the next most important source of funds for adopting hospitals, with 15% ranking the category highest. Other sources, such as the Department of Defense and private physicians, were most important for 9.5% of the adopters. State and foundation grants were the most important sources of revenue for 8% and 6.3% of the adopters, respectively. Finally, other hospital sources and affiliated hospital sources were the most important means of financing telemedicine projects for very few hospitals in the sample. None of these results reflected any geographical biases.

The information about telemedicine financing obtained from the survey is fairly straightforward. The interesting questions involve how hospital administrators plan to pay for telemedicine in the future. Hospital administrators and telemedicine project coordinators interviewed for this research held one of two viewpoints about this subject. The majority expressed vague expectations that the Health Care Financing Administration (HCFA) would ultimately reimburse for telemedical consultations, thus offsetting a large portion of the expenses.[5] Administrators in this group had not developed plans beyond continued grant monies or hopes for a change in HCFA regulations to financially sustain their telemedicine activities.

Administrators in the second, or minority, group had initiated telemedicine projects on a limited basis, offering only image-based services, such as radiology, pathology, and limited cardiology. Such projects could be financially self-supporting (in terms of operating expenses) from the outset because HCFA and other insurers already provided reimbursement for these types of consultations, which do not involve face-to-face patient encounters even without telemedicine.

The lack of certainty about future HCFA reimbursement for telemedicine is a critical issue for the financing of telemedicine. Without this reimbursement, few hospital administrators were able to identify applications of telemedicine that would make sense for their hospital. As explained above, increased managed care penetration and capitated pricing for health care may make this point obsolete. Capitated pricing regimes fundamentally change the reimbursement scenario and, therefore, change the incentives hospitals face. In such an environment, hospitals would choose to use telemedicine technologies if the technologies reduce costs, and prices or reimbursement would be irrelevant.

6.2.4   Specialties using telemedicine

Question 5 on the survey asked hospitals to indicate how frequently various medical specialties, or departments in the hospital, were using telemedicine. Table 6-9 shows the distribution the specialties that use telemedicine at least monthly (i.e., either daily, weekly, or monthly).

Table 6-9. Specialty Use of Telemedicine

Specialty	Percent of Hospitals Using Telemedicine Daily, Weekly, or Monthly
Radiology	23 (37%)
Emergency medicine	14 (22%)
Pathology	11 (17%)
Cardiology	9 (14%)
Internal medicine	7 (11%)
Pediatrics	6 (9.5%)
Psychiatry	5 (8%)
Obstetrics/gynecology	5 (8%)
Other	5 (8%)
Dermatology	4 (6%)
Surgery	4 (6%)
Urology	2 (3%)

Table 6-9 shows that radiologists use telemedicine the most. In order of use, radiology is followed by emergency medicine, pathology, cardiology, internal medicine, and pediatrics. Departments of psychiatry, obstetrics and gynecology, dermatology, surgery, and urology use the technology with decreasing frequencies. Applications of telemedicine reported in the "Other" category included dentistry, oral surgery, oncology, family practice, and geriatrics. Statistically, there was a significant bias toward urban hospitals using telemedicine for emergency medicine more frequently than rural hospitals (χ^2=9.3, p=0.002). Similarly, a bias existed toward urban hospitals using the technology for pathology more frequently than rural hospitals (χ^2=9.02, p=0.003). These were the only two specialties for which such geographic biases were statistically significant.[6]

The fact that radiology and pathology were among the most frequent users of telemedicine was not surprising in light of the fact that insurers will reimburse for these types of consultations but not for other telemedical consultations. Another explanation of the relatively high frequency with which these two specialties used telemedicine is the image-based, as opposed to "hands-on," nature of their practice. For these specialties, the adoption of telemedicine requires less change in practice routines.

6.2.5 Barriers to adoption

Question 3 in the survey helped disentangle some of the complexities of the financial and behavioral forces that explain whether a hospital will adopt telemedicine. This question probed the barriers to adopting telemedicine. Hospital administrators were asked to rank the significance of 10 potential barriers to adopting telemedicine using a Likert scale, which ranged from 1 (potential barrier was not significant) to 5 (a very significant barrier). Table 6-10 reports the results of this inquiry.

Table 6-10. Barriers to Adoption

Important Barrier (Received Score of 4 or 5 on Likert Scale)	Frequency (Percentage) of "Important" Ranking
Cost of purchasing technology	40 (64%)
Physician acceptance	32 (51%)
Cost of telecommunications	31 (49%)
Lack of insurance reimbursement	29 (46%)
Lack of industry standards	24 (38%)
Lack of internal interest or expertise	18 (29%)
Medical liability issues	17 (27%)
Patient acceptance	11 (18%)
Medical licensure issues	9 (13%)

In Table 6-10, a barrier is considered important to a hospital if it received a ranking of 4 or 5 on the Likert scale. Thus, the cost of telemedicine technology was ranked as an important barrier by 64% of hospitals. Physician acceptance was the second most frequently cited important barrier, with 51% of hospitals ranking it with a 4 or 5. These barriers were followed, in order of frequency, by the cost of telecommunications, lack of insurance reimbursement, lack of industry standards, lack of internal interest or expertise, medical liability issues, patient acceptance, and medical licensure issues.

Of the top four barriers to adopting telemedicine, three were financial issues and only one—physician acceptance—was a behavioral issue. The three financial issues were interrelated. Because many types of telemedicine consultations were not reimbursed by insurance, hospitals could not allocate the costs of telemedicine technologies or the attendant telecommunications expenses across patient visits, as they would with clinical technologies such as CT scanners. Therefore, the initial cost of purchasing telemedicine equipment proved to be an important barrier. The remaining five potential barriers merit some explanation.

Lack of industry standards refers to the fact that telemedicine equipment is not standardized. Not all equipment is compatible with other types of telemedicine equipment, making the purchase of telemedicine technologies not only expensive, but also complicated and risky. If industry standards develop or evolve, equipment that does not conform to these standards will be of limited use (OTA 1992).

Lack of internal interest is a barrier when the hospital administrator and/or the hospital staff simply have no interest in adopting telemedicine. Given the newness of the technology, it is likely that many administrators and hospital staff had never encountered information about telemedicine, with which they might form an opinion or interest.

Medical liability issues constitute a barrier to adoption if the practice of telemedicine involves greater or unforeseen medical liabilities on the part of the hospital. Since telemedicine is such a new technology, neither legal precedents nor practice guidelines currently exist to deal with liability issues.

Patient acceptance is a barrier to adoption if the administrator and/or medical practitioners believe that patients would be uncomfortable with telemedicine technologies. The risk of losing patients, or of purchasing a technology that would remain unused to avoid making patients uncomfortable, may deter adoption.

Finally, medical licensure issues would be a barrier to adoption if a telemedicine linkage crosses state borders, and the medical board of one state does not recognize the license of a physician from another state. At the time of this research, this issue was very relevant, as evidenced by recent legislation introduced in Kansas, Nevada, Oklahoma, and South Dakota, which made it illegal for physicians without a state medical license to practice telemedicine in these states (Richards 1996). These were merely the first examples of efforts to geographically restrict telemedicine practice. Policies aimed at limiting physician competition from outside the state were under consideration in at least 20 other states at the time of this research. As such initiatives become more commonplace and widely understood, this type of legislation may become an important factor in the extent and speed with which telemedicine diffuses.

These questions on the survey produced information that represents exploratory research. The answers from these questions help to complete the story told by the theory and modeling used in this research. Because this section reported exploratory research, the answers to the questions do not stand alone but must be examined in the context of the larger design and questions of this research project.

6.3 Descriptive statistics of diffusion model variables

This section provides descriptive information about the variables used in the diffusion model and compares respondents to nonrespondents to rule out or account for systematic differences between these groups. These variables come from three sources: the American Hospital Association (AHA), the 1995 Area Resource Files (ARF), and the survey.

6.3.1 Univariate analysis of market characteristic variables

This section describes the data included in the diffusion model as market characteristics. Table 6-11 describes these data.

Table 6-11. Market Characteristics Variables

Variable	Mean for Respondents	Standard Deviation for Respondents	Mean for Non-respondents	Standard Deviation for Nonrespond-ents
NEAREST	1.98	1.03	1.94	1.01
HMOPEN	2.98	6.30	3.80	6.23
POPULAT*	4.47	1.72	5.07	1.91
INCOME†	16,298	2,764	16,841	2,966

*Difference significant at the 0.002 level.
†Difference significant at the 0.10 level.

The figures in Table 6-11 show no statistically significant difference between the respondents and nonrespondents for the variables representing the natural log of the distance to the next nearest hospital (NEAREST), the percentage of the population enrolled in HMOs (HMOPEN), and per capita income (INCOME) in the county or MSA. The difference in the log of the population in the county or MSA (POPULAT) is significant at the 0.002 level; this result is to be expected, given that there was a statistically significant bias toward rural hospitals responding to the survey (Table 6-9). These results were analyzed using an independent samples *t*-test method and a one-way ANOVA between groups design. Both techniques yielded similar results.

6.3.2 Univariate analysis of hospital characteristics

This section describes the data included in the model as hospital characteristics. Tables 6-12 and 6-13 provide a summary of these variables.

Table 6-12. Hospital Characteristics: Categorical Variables

Variable	Frequency in Pop.	Percent in Pop.	Frequency Among Respond-ents	Percent of Respond-ents	χ^2 (prob) {Fisher's Exact Test: 2-tail}
RURAL*	186	53.3	100	60.2	6.13 (p=0.013) {0.014}
TEACH	19	5.46	10	6.06	0.219 (p=0.64) {0.65}
INVEST†	50	14.3	17	10.24	4.31 (p=0.04) {0.046}

*Difference significant at the 0.01 level.
†Difference significant at the 0.05 level.

Table 6-12 shows that there was a statistically significant difference between the respondents of the survey and the general population for geographic location (RURAL) and ownership structure (INVEST). Among the respondents, there were proportionally more hospitals located in rural (non-MSA) areas than in the population as a whole; in addition, there were proportionally fewer investor-owned, for-profit hospitals than in the population as a whole. The proportion of hospitals that were members of the Council of Teaching Hospitals (COTH) was representative of that in the general population.

Table 6-13. Hospital Characteristics Variables: Continuous Variables

Variable	Mean for Respondents	Standard Deviation for Respondents	Mean for Non-respondents	Standard Deviation for Non-respondents
BEDS	173.66	188.96	156.58	146.15

Using this measure of hospital size, there was no statistically significant difference in terms of size between respondents and nonrespondents. Exactly as for the market characteristics variables, these results were analyzed using an independent samples *t*-test method and a one-way ANOVA between groups design. Both techniques yielded similar results. However, these figures do not paint a very clear picture of the distribution of hospital sizes among the population and among respondents.

Table 6-14 describes the distribution of hospital sizes. The SMALLEST category of hospitals accounts for hospitals with 50 or fewer beds and corresponds to the smallest quartile (25%) of hospitals in the population. SMALL represents hospitals with between 51 and 101 beds and corresponds to the second quartile. MEDIUM represents the third quartile, hospitals with between 102 and 224 beds. BIG represents the fourth quartile of hospitals, those with over 225 beds.

Table 6-14. Hospital Size Distribution

Variable	Frequency in Pop.	Percent in Pop.	Frequency Among Respondents	Percent of Respondents	χ^2 (prob) {Fisher's Exact Test: 2-tail}
SMALL-EST*	87	24.93	50	30.12	4.56 (p=0.03) {0.036}
SMALL	88	25.21	37	22.29	1.44 (p=0.23) {0.267}
MEDIUM	87	24.93	35	21.08	2.50 (p=0.11) {0.137}
BIG	87	24.93	44	26.51	0.421 (p=0.52) {0.537}

*Difference significant at the 0.05 level.

The figures in Table 6-14 show that the smallest hospitals were proportionally overrepresented among respondents; this bias was statistically significant and was expected due to the bias toward rural hospitals responding. More importantly, Table 6-14 provides an improved picture of the ranges and distribution of the size of hospitals in the population and among respondents.

6.3.3 Univariate analysis of behavioral characteristics

This section describes the variable for measuring technological sophistication, or experience with similar technologies: TECHINDX. It also describes the variables accounting for affiliations with other hospitals.

Question 6 on the survey asked hospitals about their adoption of, or plans to adopt, information systems in three different administrative areas: inventory management, patient billing, and medical records. TECHINDX is a continuous variable constructed from survey information (section 5.4.4), which was included in the diffusion model. Table 6-15 provides the summary statistics for TECHINDX. No comparison was possible between respondents and nonrespondents because these data derive from the survey and hence were available only for respondents.[7]

Table 6-15. Technological Sophistication

Variable	Mean	Standard Deviation
TECHINDX	3.92	2.44

This information simply means that on average, hospitals responding to the survey scored 3.92 on a scale from 0 to 9 that represents technological sophistication. Table 6-16 illustrates the distribution of the TECHINDX, providing a more complete picture of technological sophistication among responding hospitals.

Table 6-16. TECHINDX Distribution

TECHINDX Score	Number of Responding Hospitals	Percentage of Responding Hospitals
9	2	1.3
8	11	7.2
7	13	8.5
6	21	13.7
5	15	9.8
4	23	15.0
3	18	11.8
2	22	14.4
1	13	8.5
0	15	9.8

Table 6-16 shows that roughly one third of the hospitals scored between 0 and 2; slightly over one third scored between 3 and 5; and the remaining one third scored 6 and over. Thus, the respondents are somewhat skewed toward the low end of the index.

Question 11 on the survey asked hospitals about their affiliations. Approximately 30% of the responding hospitals were members of multihospital systems; a clear majority of respondents (87.2%) were members of group purchasing alliances; and 37.3% were members of integrated delivery networks. Affiliation categories are not mutually exclusive. These results are summarized in Table 6-17.

Table 6-17. Affiliations with Other Hospitals

Variable	Frequency Among Respondents	Percent of Respondents
AFFILMHS	46	30.7
AFFILGPA	130	87.2
AFFILIDN	53	37.3

6.4 Conclusions

This chapter presented information that characterized the survey population and the respondents. It supplied evidence to support treating the three states as a relatively homogeneous region. The chapter described the types of hospitals that responded to the survey as well as hospitals' answers to survey questions. The answers to survey questions not specifically included in the diffusion model, in addition to the qualitative data gathered in the interviews, provide the context for further data analysis. Neither this chapter nor its constituent subsections stand on their own.

NOTES

1. The South Atlantic region consists of Delaware, Maryland, the District of Columbia, Virginia, West Virginia, North Carolina, South Carolina, Georgia, and Florida (U.S. Department of Commerce 1995).

2. For MSAs that cross state borders, the population reported reflects the population of the entire MSA, not just the portion of it in a particular state.

3. personal communication, Rebecca A. Cheatham, Telemedicine Consultant, Candler Hospital, Savannah, GA, April 20, 1995

4. As explained in Hatcher and Stepanski (1994, 169), "when analyzing a 2x2 classification table, it is best to use *Fisher's exact test* rather than the standard chi-square test of independence." Because the interpretation of this test is analogous to the chi-square test, the probability of the Fisher's exact test is reported below the chi-square analyses throughout this manuscript.

5. The Health Care Financing Administration (HCFA) sets reimbursement policies for Medicare and Medicaid. Most other insurers follow HCFA in their reimbursement policies. Currently, HCFA does not reimburse for "non–face-to-face consultations,"which include telemedicine (Smits and Baum 1995). The exceptions are for radiology and pathology consultations, which do not take place "face-to-face" under normal circumstances.

6. The small number of responses in each of the other categories may explain the lack of geographic bias in these categories. Based on these numbers, ruling out such a bias is not prudent.

7. As with the other continuous variables used in this study, the probability of this variable being normally distributed is 0.0001, using either a students-t distribution to test normality or a Shapiro-Wilk statistic. Thus, we must reject the null hypothesis that these data are distributed normally and it is reasonable to conclude that it the variable was not normally distributed.

CHAPTER 7

Data Analysis, Findings, and Discussion

This chapter reports and analyzes the results of the bivariate and multivariate analyses of factors influencing the adoption of telemedicine. While the bivariate analyses are informative, they represent exploratory rather than explanatory research: They probe relationships and suggest directions of thought. The multivariate analysis, or diffusion modeling, tells a more reliable story about the factors that influence the adoption of telemedicine. The multivariate analysis examines all the theoretically relevant relationships simultaneously, controlling for interrelationships between variables. In this chapter, the bivariate analyses are reported first, laying the groundwork for the multivariate analysis. The results of the diffusion modeling are reported next, including tests for goodness of fit. After reporting, explaining, and scrutinizing the model and the results it produced, this chapter briefly discusses these results.

7.1 Bivariate analyses

This section reports the results of simple bivariate analyses of association between the independent variables used in the diffusion model and the dependent variable, the adoption of telemedicine (Q1ANEW). Analysis of variance (ANOVA) techniques were used for identifying association between the continuous variables and adoption (Q1ANEW), and the chi-square test (with a Fisher's Exact test) was performed on the categorical variables to test for associations with adoption (Q1ANEW).

7.1.1 Relationship between market characteristics and adoption

Table 7-1 shows the means and variances of the market characteristics for both the adopters of telemedicine and the nonadopters. These results were analyzed using an independent samples *t*-test method and a one-way ANOVA between groups design. Both techniques yielded similar results: None of the market characteristics variables exhibited a statistically significant difference between adopters and nonadopters. However, the ANOVA analysis revealed a marginally significant difference between adopters and nonadopters for the variable measuring health maintenance organization (HMO) penetration, HMOPEN.

Table 7-1. Market Characteristics Variables and Telemedicine Adoption

Variable	Mean for Adopters	Standard Deviation for Adopters	Mean for Nonadopters	Standard Deviation for Nonadopters
NEAREST	1.8531	1.0823	2.0650	0.9828
HMOPEN	0.03984	0.07119	0.02316	0.05631
POPULAT *	4.8099	1.6084	4.2414	1.7689
INCOME	16,698	2,904	16,032	2,649

*Significant at 0.05 level in ANOVA analysis.

7.1.2 Relationship between hospital characteristics and adoption

Table 7-2 shows the distribution of the hospital characteristics variables in the respondents as a whole and the distribution among adopters. A chi-square test and a Fisher's Exact test probed the bivariate relationship between the dependent variable, adoption of telemedicine, and the hospital characteristics.

Table 7-2. Hospital Characteristics and Telemedicine Adoption: Categorical Variables

Variable	Frequency Among Respond-ents	Percent Among Respond-ents	Frequency Among Adopters	Percent of Adopters	χ^2 (prob) {Fisher's Exact Test: 2-tail}
RURAL *	98	60.9	32	48.5	6.33 (p=0.01) {0.015}
TEACH †	10	6.06	7	10.61	3.992 (p=0.05) {0.091}
INVEST *	17	10.24	2	3.03	6.19 (p=0.01) {0.017}

*Difference significant at the 0.01 level.
†Difference significant at the 0.05 level.

The significance of the chi-square (and Fisher's Exact) statistics suggested that a relationship exists between adoption of telemedicine and the characteristics of location (RURAL), teaching status (TEACH), and ownership status[1] (INVEST). These analyses suggested a negative relationship between a hospital's location in a rural area, as well as for-profit status, and adoption. They also suggested a positive relationship between teaching status and adoption.

Table 7-3 provides the summary statistics of the bivariate analysis of the relationship between hospital size (BEDS) and adoption of telemedicine.

Table 7-3. Bivariate Association Between Hospital Size and Adoption

Variable	Mean for Adopters	Standard Deviation for Adopters	Mean for Nonadopters	Standard Deviation for Nonadopters
BEDS*	235.36	228.08	132.93	145.41

*Difference significant at the 0.01 level.

This analysis showed a statistically significant difference between adopters and nonadopters in terms of their mean size. Hospitals that adopted telemedicine were statistically significantly larger than nonadopters. As for the market characteristics variables, these results were analyzed using an independent samples t-test method and a one-way ANOVA between groups design. Both techniques yielded similar results.

7.1.3 Relationship between behavioral characteristics and adoption

Table 7-4 provides the summary statistics of the bivariate analysis of the relationship between technological sophistication (TECHINDX) and the adoption of telemedicine.

Table 7-4. Bivariate Association Between Technological Sophistication and Adoption

Variable	Mean for Adopters	Standard Deviation for Adopters	Mean for Non-adopters	Standard Deviation for Non-adopters
TECHINDX*	4.41	2.69	3.61	2.22

*Difference significant at the 0.05 level.

When examined in isolation from other effects, the difference in the mean of technological sophistication between adopters and nonadopters was statistically significant. Hospitals that adopted telemedicine were statistically significantly more technologically sophisticated, or had implemented more information technologies, than nonadopters. Exactly as for the market characteristics variables, these results were analyzed using an independent samples *t*-test method and a one-way ANOVA between groups design. Both techniques yielded similar results.

Table 7-5 summarizes the bivariate associations between the variables representing affiliations and the adoption of telemedicine.

Table 7-5. Bivariate Association Between Affiliations and Adoption

Variable	Frequency Among Respond-ents	Percent Among Respond-ents	Frequency Among Adopters	Percent of Adopters	χ^2 (prob) {Fisher's Exact Test: 2-tail}
AFFIL-MHS	46	30. 7	19	32.76	0.19 (p=0.66) {0.72}
AFFIL-GPA	130	87.2	53	91.38	1.457 (p=0.23) {0.32}
AFFIL-IDN*	53	37.3	28	49.12	5.667 (p=0.02) {0.02}

*Difference significant at the 0.05 level.

Table 7-5 shows no significant bivariate relationship between two of the hospital characteristics (AFFILMHS, AFFILGPA) and whether a hospital adopts telemedicine. This result suggests that neither affiliation in a multihospital system nor affiliation in a group purchasing alliance influences the probability of adopting telemedicine. The relationship between affiliation in an integrated delivery network (AFFILIDN) and adoption was significant at the 0.05 level, suggesting that there may be a relationship between this particular type of hospital affiliation and telemedicine adoption.

7.2 Multivariate analysis: The diffusion model

This section reports the results of the diffusion model, assesses the model's goodness of fit, and interprets these results. Of course, the multivariate analysis is only as reliable as the specification of the model. The diffusion model derives directly from economic and sociological models of the diffusion of innovations. No a priori or theoretical reasoning existed to suggest relationships other than additive, direct effects from the independent variables on the dependent variable. Therefore, the model presented is very straightforward in its specification.

7.2.1 Results of the diffusion model

Table 7-6 provides a summary of the parameter estimates, their standard errors, the chi-square statistic and the probability value (p-value) of the chi-square statistic, the odds ratios, and their confidence intervals. The variables indicated with one asterisk were statistically significant at the 0.10 level; those indicated with a dagger were significant at the 0.05 level.

Table 7-6. Diffusion Model Results

Variable	Parameter Estimate (Standard Error)	χ^2 (prob)	Odds Ratio	Wald Confidence Limits for Odds Ratio: Lower-Upper Bounds
INTERCEPT	-6.02 (2.56)	5.54 (0.02)	Not Applicable	Not Applicable
NEAREST	0.26 (0.27)	0.92 (0.34)	1.3	0.76 2.22
HMOPEN	0.015 (0.055)	0.08 (0.78)	1.01	0.91 1.13
POPULAT	-0.27 (0.31)	0.76 (0.38)	0.76	0.4 1.41
INCOME	0.005 (0.014)	0.16 (0.69)	1.00	0.98 1.03

RURAL	-1.03	1.84	0.36	0.08
	(0.76)	(0.17)		1.58
TEACH	-0.13	0.01	0.88	0.09
	(1.14)	(0.91)		8.28
NOTPROFT†	2.11	4.60	8.24	1.20
	(0.98)	(0.03)		56.61
BEDS*	0.53	2.77	1.70	0.91
	(0.32)	(0.096)		3.19
AFFILMHS†	1.13	4.18	3.09	1.05
	(0.55)	(0.04)		9.09
AFFILGPA	0.84	1.09	2.32	0.48
	(0.81)	(0.29)		11.30
AFFILIDN*	0.82	3.52	2.28	0.97
	(0.44)	(0.06)		5.37
TECHINDX	0.05	0.30	1.05	0.87
	(0.09)	(0.58)		1.27

*Significant at 0.10 level.

†Significant at 0.05 level.

By several measures, the described model fits the data well. The log likelihood test statistic (-2LogL) had a chi-square value of 24.73, with 12 degrees of freedom and a probability of 0.016. This test is analogous to the F test of the joint significance of the independent variables from ordinary least squares (OLS) regression (Stokes, Davis, and Koch 1995). It is interpreted to mean that a probability of 0.016 exists that all of the parameter estimates (the β's) are truly equal to zero, a sufficiently low probability to indicate that the model fits the data adequately. Additional indicators of goodness of fit: The model correctly predicted 71.8% of the responses; the pseudo-R^2=25%, a value comparable to similar models in the literature.[2]

Several diagnostic tests were run to assess the strength of the model because the diagnostics for logistic regressions are much less developed than those for OLS regression (Stokes, Davis, and Koch 1995). Although these tests generated somewhat conflicting results, they suggested there might be multicollinearity between the variables representing rural location, teaching status, size of the population of the hospital's county or MSA, the log of the distance to the next closest hospital, HMO penetration, per capita income, size of the hospital, and technological sophistication (RURAL, TEACH, POPULAT, NEAREST, HMOPEN, INCOME, BEDS, and TECHINDX, respectively). This possibility would make interpreting the coefficients and odds ratios that correspond to these variables difficult. Since these variables are all related to the geographic dichotomy of urban and rural locations, they will be referred to henceforth as the category of GEOGRAPHY variables. After exploring and implementing alternative methods of analysis to correct for the problems with the data, the initial model remained the best, and is reported with the attendant caveats.

The model shows that not-for-profit (NFP) status, hospital size, affiliation with a multihospital system, and affiliation with an integrated delivery network (NOTPROFT, BEDS, AFFILMHS, and AFFILIDN, respectively) were statistically significant variables predicting the adoption of telemedicine. NFP status and affiliation with a multihospital system (NOTPROFT and AFFILMHS) were significant at the 0.05 level; size and affiliation with an integrated delivery network (BEDS and AFFILIDN) were significant at the 0.10 level. These results predicted that an NFP hospital was approximately 8.2 times as likely as an investor-owned (IO) hospital to adopt telemedicine. Hospitals that are members of multihospital systems were roughly 3 times as likely as independent hospitals to adopt telemedicine. An increase in a log-transformed unit of beds increased the odds of adoption by a factor of 1.7; this means that larger hospitals were more likely than smaller hospitals to adopt telemedicine. Members of integrated delivery networks (IDNs) were slightly over 2 times as likely as unaffiliated hospitals to adopt telemedicine.

7.2.2 Getting beneath the surface of the model results

Before relating these results to the hypotheses proposed in chapter 4, further examination of the model is warranted. Not coincidentally, three of the four variables that exhibit no interdependence with the class of GEOGRAPHY variables had statistical significance in the model. Only one of the remaining variables was statistically significant. While the bivariate analyses (section 7.1) suggested that several of the GEOGRAPHY variables would be related to telemedicine adoption, the fact that they are so interrelated confounded the interpretation of their precise effects on the adoption of telemedicine.

The associations among the GEOGRAPHY variables were not unexpected. First, rural areas are, by definition, less populated than urban areas, which explains the relationship between rural location and population (RURAL and POPULAT). Further, smaller hospitals are typically located in less populated areas because fewer hospital beds are necessary; thus, the relationship between size, rural location, and population. Similarly, fewer hospitals are located in any given rural community due to the low population and high fixed cost of building and operating a hospital; thus, the variable representing distance to the next closest hospital (NEAREST) is also related to geography and population. HMO development has been a largely urban phenomenon, and this fact is no different in the region of study. Finally, technological sophistication (TECHINDX) was the only independent variable in this category of interrelated variables that would not necessarily belong in this group. Although it is not surprising that rural hospitals, which are typically smaller and possess fewer financial and personnel resources, would use fewer information technologies,[3] it is not unreasonable to assume that this variable would be neutral with respect to geography. Because these variables are so mutually dependent, when they were included together in a multivariate analysis, disentangling their independent effects was nearly impossible.

Among the standard approaches to correcting for multicollinearity is principal components analysis. Although this technique was used, it did not improve the explanatory power of the model. The most intuitive technique for dealing with multicollinearity is to eliminate at least one of the multicollinear variables. Even though this method introduces left-out variable bias and diminishes the explanatory power of the model, it is instructive. This process was undertaken methodically by first eliminating one variable at a time, then eliminating the class of interrelated variables, and including each variable by itself. Dropping any one of these interrelated variables did not produce greater significance among the remaining independent variables in the group. The process of eliminating all of the GEOGRAPHY variables except one, then sequentially introducing a single variable from this category produced the most interesting and revealing results. By the -2LogL criterion, each of the reduced form models fit the data better than the fully specified model; however, this was partially an artifact of having fewer degrees of freedom. In addition, each of the reduced form models improved the explanatory power of the model over that of the model with none of the GEOGRAPHY variables. The pseudo-R^2 values of the reduced form models were all lower than those of the fully specified model. This statistic is most useful in comparing the relative fit of the reduced form models because the psuedo-R^2 accounts for the increased number of explanatory variables in the fully specified model.

On balance, four of the GEOGRAPHY variables provide impressive explanatory power within the reduced form model. The reduced form model with the BEDS variable calculated that the odds of adopting telemedicine increased by 60% with the addition of each logged-transformed unit of beds. Therefore, this model suggested that the adoption of telemedicine was positively associated with hospital size. This model also confirmed that NFP status and affiliation with an integrated delivery network (NOTPROFT and AFFILIDN) each increased the odds of adopting by factors of approximately 6.0 and 2.0, respectively. This result was consistent with the fully specified model.

By substituting the variable measuring the population of the hospital's county or MSA (POPULAT) for the class of interrelated variables, the model predicted an increase of 20% in the odds of adopting telemedicine for each additional log-transformed unit of 1000 in population. This model, therefore, suggested that adoption of telemedicine was positively related to community size. Again, the variables representing ownership status and membership in an integrated delivery network (IDN) remained strong positive influences in the odds of adoption in this model, with odds ratios of 6.53 and 2.25, respectively.

When the variable denoting rural location (RURAL) was substituted into the model, the odds ratio was 0.47. This means that hospitals located outside an MSA are approximately one half as likely to adopt telemedicine as hospitals located in an MSA; in other words, urban hospitals were nearly twice as likely to adopt telemedicine as rural hospitals. Again, the variables for NFP status and affiliation with an IDN were statistically significant in this reduced form model, increasing the odds of adoption by factors of 7.2 and 2.1, respectively.

The comparison of the simplified models demonstrated that among the GEOGRAPHY variables, hospital size and community location (BEDS and RURAL) exert the strongest effect on adoption: None of the other GEOGRAPHY characteristics proved significant while also achieving adequate model fit. These two variables are obviously quite interdependent and separating their individual effects was not possible with this data set. These results did not rule out the possibility that the other GEOGRAPHY variables might independently influence adoption. The fact that the group of GEOGRAPHY variables was interrelated certainly confounded the interpretation of the multivariate analysis. It did, however, suggest that rural or urban location are not defined simply by geography or population, but rather are multidimensional concepts.

The results from the comparison of reduced form models established a relationship between hospital size or community location and telemedicine adoption. Although the precise nature of this relationship remained clouded, the exercise elucidated a positive effect that was masked by the multicollinearity of the GEOGRAPHY variables included in the fully specified model. This comparison also illustrated the robustness of the findings from the fully specified model that ownership status and affiliations (NOTPROFT, AFFILIDN, and AFFILMHS) strongly and positively influenced telemedicine adoption. These results were consistent in magnitude and direction across all variations of the diffusion model.

7.3 Summary of bivariate and multivariate analyses

Although bivariate analyses are often considered exploratory research, the analyses presented in section 7.1 served an important analytic purpose in this chapter. They provided a reference point for the multivariate analyses. The bivariate analyses suggested a positive relationship between the adoption of telemedicine and the variables measuring population, hospital size, technological sophistication, rural location, teaching status, ownership status, and affiliation in an integrated delivery network (IDN). The fully specified diffusion model clarified the strength of the positive associations between ownership status, affiliations, and adoption. In this analysis, the spurious associations between adoption and several of the independent variables, which were significant in bivariate analyses, were shown to be insignificant: artifacts more of the associations among the independent variables than of true relationships with the dependent variable. Finally, the comparison of reduced form diffusion models helped to identify the specific qualities of urban location—hospital and community size—that were related to telemedicine adoption and were suggested by the bivariate analyses. These tests of reduced form models also provided support for the findings from the fully specified model. In each version of the models, NFP status and affiliations with other hospitals significantly increased the odds of adopting telemedicine. The fact that ownership status and affiliations remained consistently positive and significant in predicting telemedicine adoption across both the fully specified model and the various reduced form models demonstrated the robustness of these findings. The next chapter discusses these findings and their significance relative to the hypotheses and to policy issues.

NOTES

1. Due to the small number of investor-owned hospitals that adopted telemedicine (2), the chi-square test of this association can be unreliable.

2. The pseudo-R2 is calculated as ESS/(ESS+3.29*N), where ESS is the explained sum of squares and N is the total sample size. This calculation follows the technique described in Aldrich and Nelson (1984). As a comparison, Tepelensky et al. report a pseudo-R2 of 5% (although their calculation is somewhat different). If the model offers no improvement over a restricted model, with all the parameters set to zero, the pseudo-R2 will be zero; if the model perfectly describes the observations, the pseudo-R2 will approach one. The main difficulty with this measure of fit is that it "does not incorporate a penalty for increasing the number of exogenous variables," nor is it universally accepted or used (Aldrich and Nelson 1984).

3. In fact, location theory would predict this result.

Conclusions and Policy Implications

This final chapter summarizes the theoretical and empirical research presented in the earlier chapters. The findings from the qualitative and quantitative empirical research to the hypotheses posed in chapter 4 are compared. After relating this research to the hypotheses, the chapter applies the findings to the larger policy context. Finally, chapter 8 discusses the limitations of this study and offers directions for future research.

8.1 Empirical research and hypothesis testing

The original purpose of this research was to investigate whether and how telemedicine influences hospitals' costs. By determining whether telemedicine generates internalizable cost savings for hospitals, the research would have documented one type of benefit that these technologies may confer. This information, in combination with other studies about the potential health care benefits of these technologies, could be compared to the costs—both to hospitals and government organizations—of implementing and utilizing telemedicine. A cost-benefit analysis of this type would help clarify the appropriate role for government in developing telemedicine and information infrastructure technologies.

The necessary data to carry out the cost-benefit analysis were unobtainable, and in many cases, intractable due to the complex and multiple financing arrangements for telemedicine within and across individual hospitals. As a result, the goals of this research were reassessed and the empirical components of this research were redirected to take into account the paucity of data about this very interesting and policy-driven subject. Accordingly, the objective of this research evolved into a study of how telemedicine is diffusing in its early stages of development. By understanding what the characteristics of adopters implied about the potential and actual benefits these technologies offer, it would be possible to make plausible inferences to answer the same types of questions originally posed. Therefore, the modified objectives of this research were (1) to identify characteristics and economic environments of hospitals that are related to adopting telemedicine technologies, (2) to make reasonable and informed inferences about the types of benefits hospitals can derive from these technologies, using theory, quantitative research, and qualitative research, and (3) to relate these findings back to current policy objectives to identify feasible, appropriate roles for government in developing telemedicine.

To reiterate the findings from chapters 6 and 7, the results of the quantitative analyses reveal that each of the following factors independently increase the odds of adopting telemedicine: not-for-profit (NFP) status (NOTPROFT); affiliation with a multihospital system (AFFILMHS); affiliation with an integrated delivery network (AFFILIDN); and characteristics of urban location—most prominently, larger hospital size (BEDS). Thus, NFP hospitals are much more likely to adopt telemedicine than are investor-owned (IO) hospitals; telemedicine is more attractive for hospitals that are members of integrated delivery networks or multihospital systems. The fact that larger hospitals are more likely to adopt telemedicine suggests that some form of economies of scale is involved with the decision to adoption of telemedicine. These results are summarized in Table 8-1.

Table 8-1. Factors Increasing the Odds of Telemedicine Adoption

Characteristic	Increase in Odds of Adoption
Not-for-profit (NFP) status	7.5
Affiliation in an integrated delivery network (IDN)	2.3
Affiliation in a multihospital system (MHS)	2.6
Hospital size (measured in log-transformed units of beds)	1.60

The qualitative research from the survey suggested that telemedicine plays an important role in hospitals' plans for competitiveness and adaptation to managed care, although quantitative evidence to support this conclusion was less convincing. In the diffusion model, penetration by health maintenance organizations (HMOs) was not a significant predictor of telemedicine adoption nor was competitiveness of the local hospital's market, as measured by distance to the next closest hospital. The interviews indicated that hospital administrators had not necessarily adopted telemedicine with a managed care strategy in mind. Nonetheless, administrators invariably could envision ways that telemedicine could prove profitable in a capitated pricing environment, where there are great incentives to keep patients out of the hospital—particularly expensive tertiary care centers. Finally, technological sophistication, measured by an index of other information technologies used by a hospital, surprisingly proved to be unrelated with adopting telemedicine technologies. This finding, and further explorations of the concept of technological sophistication, indicated that larger hospitals tended to have more hospital information system technologies. However, greater technological sophistication was not a precursor to the adoption of telemedicine; instead, technological sophistication appeared to be a function of scale economies.

These results are discussed in the context of the hypotheses proposed in chapter 4. The primary hypotheses of chapter 4 frame this section. Each subsection synthesizes the results from the empirical and qualitative research and relates these results to a particular hypothesis that was identified earlier.

8.1.1 Hospital location and telemedicine adoption: H1, H1a, and H1b

Hypothesis 1. This hypothesis was critical in assessing the effectiveness of current federal and state policies promoting telemedicine as a partial solution to persistent rural health problems. The results of the modeling process provided qualified support for the primary hypothesis, H1, that hospital location is a factor in predicting telemedicine adoption. The RURAL variable was not statistically significant in the fully specified model; however, the RURAL variable was statistically significant in the reduced form model. This significance, combined with information gathered from the diagnostics performed on the fully specified model, clearly illustrated that several factors, which are virtually inseparable from urban or rural location, are positively related to telemedicine adoption. Thus, rural location is negatively related to telemedicine adoption.

The negative relationship of rural location to adoption conforms to location theory, which defines the cluster of factors that favor urban areas in terms of innovation diffusion and economic development as agglomeration economies (Isard 1956, Jacobs 1984, Maleki 1991). The existence of these agglomeration economies at least partially explains why rural location and factors, such as hospital size, population, and income of the hospital market, are statistically significant as predictors of telemedicine adoption in bivariate analyses but become insignificant in multivariate analyses. In the bivariate tests, identifying the independent effect of any given geographic attribute that is correlated with other variables is impossible. Thus, each variable represents the influence of the related variables as well. In a multivariate analysis, which better controls for the independent effect of each variable, none of these variables was a strong predictor of adoption independently. Location theory would suggest this outcome: Although location alone cannot explain telemedicine adoption, the combination of several facets of geographic location translate to a disadvantage for rural communities in gaining access to these technologies.

Hypothesis 1a. This hypothesis probed the nature of the rural disadvantage. The analyses revealed strong evidence supporting the subsidiary hypothesis, H1a, that larger hospitals are more likely to adopt telemedicine. The BEDS variable was statistically significant at the 0.10

level in the fully specified model. When tested in a reduced form model, the BEDS variable provided adequate explanatory power and was statistically significant (p=0.02). In the strictest analysis, the effects of hospital size cannot reliably be separated from the effects of community location (RURAL). Both variables produced satisfactory model fit when included independently from the other GEOGRAPHY variables in reduced form diffusion models. Both variables were statistically significant in these models, and both are strongly related to each other. However, two reasons support the conclusion that hospital size is the relevant variable that is positively associated with telemedicine adoption. First, the relative strength, measured by the -2LogL or by the pseudo-R^2 values, of the reduced form model with BEDS included was slightly greater than the reduced form model with RURAL included. Second, hospitals were the unit of analysis and the decision-making unit relative to these technologies. It simply makes sense that this factor would exert a more direct influence on technology adoption, holding all other factors equal, than would the location of the community per se. Although several factors, such as population, competition in the market, HMO penetration, and income, are positively related to location in a county or metropolitan statistical area (MSA), the direct effect of location by itself is tenuous. The fact that size of the hospital increased the likelihood of adoption is also consistent with an explanation presented by Rose and Joskow (1990)[1]: "New technologies will be relatively disadvantaged when they are embodied in indivisible capital goods, particularly if capital costs of new plants are high relative to the operating costs of existing facilities." In other words, the innovation will be less attractive when the cost of an innovation is expensive relative to the operating costs of a particular firm, as telemedicine is for smaller hospitals. Consequently, the quantitative analysis in combination with sensible logic support the hypothesis that larger hospitals are more likely to adopt telemedicine, and economies of scale exist with respect to telemedicine adoption.

Hypothesis 1b. This subsidiary hypothesis represented another exploration of factors associated with location. The empirical research provided no support for the subsidiary hypothesis, H1b, that technological sophistication is positively related with the adoption of telemedicine. None of the diffusion models foun TECHINDX to be a statistically significant variable. When included as the sole GEOGRAPHY variable in a reduced form diffusion model, TECHINDX substantially improved the model's explanatory power over that of a model without a GEOGRAPHY variable; however, the variable itself remained insignificant. At best, TECHINDX is inseparable from other characteristics of urban location or hospital size that are positively associated with telemedicine adoption.

The conclusion that technological sophistication is unrelated to telemedicine adoption is counterintuitive since telemedicine represents a very sophisticated technology. One plausible explanation, supported by statistical analyses described in chapter 7, is that the adoption of the information technologies that comprise TECHINDX is strongly and positively related to hospital size. As the size of the hospital increases, the imperative to adopt information technologies increases. Thus, the influence of technological sophistication on adoption of telemedicine is overwhelmed by the influence of hospital size.

This finding contradicts the expectations derived from theory and common sense. As Rogers (1983) explains, previous exposure to or familiarity with similar innovations generally creates a predisposition to be receptive to a related innovation. Because many of the technologies for hospital information systems rely on very similar technological components and expertise, it is somewhat surprising to find no relationship between the measure of technological sophistication and the adoption of telemedicine. Perhaps this is best explained by the fact that the constituent technologies of the TECHINDX have primarily administrative applications, whereas telemedicine is a distinctly clinical application of telecommunications and information technologies.

8.1.2 Ownership status and telemedicine adoption: H2

This hypothesis explored the existence of public- or private-type benefits derived from telemedicine, which might be reflected in differential patterns of adoption between IO and NFP hospitals. The model clearly supported the hypothesis, H2, that ownership structure plays a role in telemedicine adoption. In the fully specified diffusion model, and in each of the reduced form models, NOTPROFT was statistically significant, increasing the odds of adopting telemedicine by roughly 7.5 times. The diffusion modeling used in this research revealed an effect that was robust to model specification. This finding is partially explained by the fact that federal and state grant programs are important sources of funds for telemedicine investments, and IO hospitals are ineligible to apply for many of the grant programs.[2] Such ineligibility does not apply across all grant programs and, thus, is not a very powerful explanation.

Although the majority (38%) of responding hospitals listed operating revenues as the most important source of funds for telemedicine investments, federal and state government funds possibly constitute a threshold level of capital. This level would make investing in telemedicine financially feasible for NFP hospitals. With the cushion of government grants, NFP hospitals may be more willing or able to accept the risks involved with telemedicine, given that little is known about its financial payback. The possibility also exists that NFP hospitals are simply more willing to accept the risks entailed in investing in telemedicine because they are not as constrained by profit motives as IO hospitals. This point was well articulated by one administrator of an NFP hospital. He stated, "telemedicine is something my hospital does to serve part of its mission; as a not-for-profit, my mission is significantly different than that of an investor-owned hospital. Nobody knows the rate of return for telemedicine. Without that information, an investor-owned hospital will not make the investment." Grant funds may simply reduce the risk of investment, or NFP hospitals may behave differently from IO hospitals due to their broader mission. In either case, this research clearly demonstrates that NFP hospitals are much more likely to adopt telemedicine than IO hospitals.

This finding makes an interesting contribution to the long-standing debate in the literature about the role of ownership structure and hospital behavior. Both economic theory and empirical research provide equivocal evidence about this subject. Several researchers have demonstrated no difference in the behavior of NFP and IO hospitals (Sloan and Vraicu 1983; Friedman and Shortell 1988; Kralewski, Gifford, and Porter 1988), while others have shown such differences to exist (Alexander and Lewis 1984, Sear 1991). The strong difference between the behavior of NFP and IO hospitals demonstrated in this research may be unique to telemedicine adoption and the early stage of the development of this technology.

Nonetheless, the finding that NFP hospitals are overwhelmingly more likely than IO hospitals to be early adopters of telemedicine is interesting.

8.1.3 The strategic role of telemedicine: H3, H3a, H3b

Hypothesis 3. This hypothesis explored the nature and extent of private or internalizable benefits that telemedicine may confer. The evidence from the research produced conflicting results. The first proposed test of the primary hypothesis, H3, that telemedicine is an important technology for hospitals' competitiveness, produced no evidence. Specifically, the variable measuring distance to the nearest hospital—a proxy for competition in the local market—was statistically significant in none of the models. While it could be argued that in the fully specified model, this variable was so highly correlated with the other GEOGRAPHY variables that its effects may have been masked; when included independently in a reduced form model, it still was not significant. The fact that the inclusion of this variable in a reduced form equation was an improvement over the reduced model with none of the GEOGRAPHY variables is best explained by concluding that the NEAREST variable represents characteristics associated with urban location.

The qualitative component of this research lent a different perspective to the question posed in hypothesis H3. Questions 1b, 1d, 1e, and 1f on the hospital survey asked hospital administrators to rank, on a scale from 1 to 5, the importance of telemedicine to four aspects of the hospital's competitive strategy: adapting to a managed care environment, price competitiveness, technological leadership, and providing quality health care. Of the telemedicine adopters, 63% indicated that telemedicine was highly important to their managed care strategy. In addition, 69% of the adopters, who indicated they faced competition in their local market, reported that telemedicine was highly important to their role as a technological leader in that market. Based on this summary of qualitative responses from the survey, it was reasonable to infer that administrators foresee telemedicine playing a role in their future competitiveness in the future. The interviews with hospital administrators confirmed this conclusion. When questioned as to why their hospital had adopted telemedicine, the most commonly cited reason was for marketing purposes. The term "positioning," summarized one administrator's perspective on the role of telemedicine in his hospital. This characterization of telemedicine reflected the comments of many of the administrators interviewed, indicating that telemedicine confers competitive advantage in terms of the hospital being perceived as innovative and state of the art. Several other administrators indicated a sense of technological inevitability about telemedicine: They had to adopt it in order to be perceived as up to date by patients and physicians.

The perception that hospital administrators considered telemedicine to be a competitive marketing tool reflects the kind of nonprice competition among hospitals that has been characterized as the "medical arms race" (Weisbrod 1991). Because consumers of medical services are often insensitive to price effects due to insurance arrangements and differences between medical services and commodity products, hospitals compete for patients on the basis of perceived quality of care as represented by amenities offered by the hospital (Robinson and Luft 1987). This explains comments of the administrator who explained that "patients see this stuff on TV and want to know that their hospital has these technologies." Similarly, hospitals compete for physician affiliations and, hence, admissions based on the "provision of services that physicians appreciate" (Robinson and Luft 1987). This type of behavior may be at work when a hospital adopts teleradiology equipment so that the local radiologist can interpret radiologic studies from his or her home.

The fact that the marketing function was identified as the most prominent strategic role for telemedicine also illustrates the power with which this technology captures the imagination of hospital administrators, patients, and physicians. Quality of care or financial advantages were rarely mentioned in interviews, likely reflecting the newness of the technologies and the attendant uncertainty about these factors. Medical efficacy and cost issues were not even close to resolution at the time of this research; in fact, the questions were still being formulated.

Hypothesis 3a: This hypothesis was very important for two reasons: First, affiliations between hospitals are widely thought to be a precursor to increased managed care penetration (Cave 1995; Curran and O'Connor 1995; Hospitals and Health Networks 1995; Kripke Byers and Levi-Baumgarten 1995; Nurkin 1995; Shortell, Gillies, and Devers 1995); thus, if telemedicine adoption is associated with membership in affiliations, then it may be an important component of an evolving strategy to compete in a managed care environment. Second, affiliations between hospitals have come to the attention of the Department of Justice and the Federal Trade Commission because of antitrust concerns. To the extent that telemedicine depends on and facilitates affiliations, it may play a central role in this policy debate.

Each of the diffusion models reported in chapter 7 supported hypothesis H3a: Affiliation with other hospitals or health care organizations is positively related to the adoption of telemedicine. The models clearly showed that affiliation with an integrated delivery network (IDN) increases the odds of adopting telemedicine by a factor of at least 2. This result held across the fully specified and each of the reduced form models. In the fully specified model, affiliation with a multihospital system (MHS) more than doubled the odds of adopting telemedicine, but in only one of the reduced form models was affiliation with a MHS significant. MHS affiliation was not as stable as the IDN variable across models; nor was it statistically significant at the 0.05 level in the fully specified model. Caution is warranted, therefore, before concluding that membership in a multihospital system increases the odds of adopting telemedicine.

These results confirmed the theoretical, commonsense notion that affiliations or network relationships provide important institutional connections, channels of communication, and applications for the use of telemedicine (McKinney 1991). More interesting, affiliation relationships may also improve hospitals' access to capital, providing another source of funds with which to invest in telemedicine (Shortell, Gillies, and Devers 1995). Affiliation with a group purchasing alliance (AFFILGPA) was not statistically significant in any of the models; thus, it was reasonable to conclude that this affiliation plays no role in telemedicine adoption.

Hypothesis 3b. This hypothesis probed whether HMO penetration and telemedicine adoption were directly associated, which is a very specific aspect of the role of telemedicine in competitive strategy. The quantitative analyses provided no support for the hypothesis, H3b, that HMO penetration would be related to telemedicine adoption. The HMOPEN variable was not statistically significant in either the fully specified diffusion model or the reduced form model. To the extent that HMO penetration is positively related with other qualities of urban location, this variable may be an unmeasured factor in telemedicine adoption. No direct, quantitative support for the influence of this factor on telemedicine adoption was revealed.

This finding was not surprising, given the low rate of HMO enrollment in the region. In the urban areas of the survey region, enrollment in federally licensed HMOs averaged 7% in 1995; in the rural areas, HMO enrollment was effectively zero.[3] Managed care was not yet a powerful enough phenomenon in this region of the United States to determine whether and how it might influence telemedicine development.

The interviews with hospital administrators provided interesting insight into the future role of telemedicine, when managed care will be a more immediate concern in this region. Several administrators explained ways in which telemedicine could be used to allow patients to stay in their community hospital or out of the hospital altogether. In a capitated pricing environment focused on patient management, a critical component of minimizing costs is the ability to appropriately determine who should be admitted and who can avoid a hospital stay. To the extent that telemedicine augments the information base used by health care providers to make such decisions, it could become a particularly important tool in a market dominated by managed care.

8.1.4 Conclusions from the hypotheses

The qualitative and quantitative analyses provided convincing evidence to support the hypotheses that hospital size, ownership structure, and strategic affiliations influence telemedicine adoption. This research found that larger hospitals are more likely than smaller hospitals to adopt telemedicine; not-for-profit hospitals are several times more likely than investor owned hospitals to adopt telemedicine; and hospitals affiliated with multihospital systems (MHS) and/or integrated delivery networks (IDNs) are at least twice as likely as nonaffiliated hospitals to adopt telemedicine. The research uncovered qualified support for the hypotheses that location and competitive strategy are factors in the adoption of telemedicine. When the quantitative evidence was inconclusive, the qualitative components strongly suggested that these factors were, indeed, important. Neither the quantitative nor the qualitative methods could support the remaining hypothesis, H1b: Technological sophistication positively influences adoption. The lack of evidence partially reflects the interrelationship between this variable and other aspects of urban location, making it difficult to separate the effects of technological sophistication from these other factors.

8.2 Beyond hypotheses: Implications for rural hospitals and policy makers

The findings of this research represent a critical first step in understanding the "second wave" of telemedicine diffusion. From a policy perspective, one of the most important findings from this research became clear before the analyses were started: Information about how these technologies affect hospital costs was unavailable for research and largely unavailable to hospital administrators investing in telemedicine in the mid 1990s. As described in chapter 2, the financing and implementation of telemedicine projects were complex. Oftentimes, financing and implementation involved several departments within one hospital, various grant and operating funds, and managers who knew little about other telemedicine activities within one institution. This scenario did not necessarily represent poor management; rather, it reflected the newness of the technologies.

With little consensus about medical efficacy and appropriate medical applications of telemedicine, no information about how telemedicine affects hospital costs, and no uniform reimbursement policies, telemedicine investments represented considerable risks in terms of capital and personnel investments. As such, it was not surprising that these technologies were being adopted on almost an experimental basis by innovative hospitals or individuals within innovative departments of hospitals.

This study provided a profile of the types of hospitals adopting telemedicine in the Southeastern US in the mid 1990s. In the absence of financial data, hospital profiles allowed for inferences to be made as to the reasons for adopting telemedicine. Figure 8-1 illustrates the configuration of telemedicine networks in North Carolina and presents a visual representation of the major findings of the empirical work.

Figure 8-1. Configuration of Telemedicine Networks in North Carolina

Figure 8-1

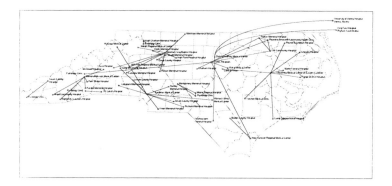

Figure 8-1 shows the hub-and-spoke structure of North Carolina's telemedicine networks. Hubs were located in the major metropolitan regions of the state; spokes were located in outlying, but rarely rural, areas.[4] Visualizing the geographic range of these networks is also interesting. At the time of this research, the state's major hospitals, or hubs, had not affiliated with outlying hospitals, or spokes, in a way that would greatly infringe or compete with each others' networks. As can be seen, this relationship was not strictly the case in the western part of the state. Although worthy of further investigation, such research was beyond the scope and resources of this project.

8.2.1 Size and location

The tendency for large hospitals in urban locations to be more likely to adopt telemedicine is strong evidence that telemedicine is not reaching rural areas. This tendency may be explained by the smaller size of rural hospitals—and smaller financial, technical, and personnel resources—or may be the result of other factors related to rural location. Nonetheless, small, rural hospitals were not participating in telemedicine initiatives at the rate of large, urban hospitals at the time of this research. Since improving rural health is the stated goal of many federal and state telemedicine grant programs, this research suggests that these programs are falling short of this goal. If federal and state governments aim to promote telemedicine as a technology to improve rural health and the viability of rural hospitals, these programs need to better target these small, rural hospitals.

Chapter 6 described the barriers to adoption reported by telemedicine adopters. In brief, the most important barrier was cost, followed by physician acceptance, lack of reimbursement, and lack of internal expertise. Small, rural hospitals are likely to face these same barriers but are unable to overcome them. Assistance in gaining access to investment capital for telemedicine, either through private or public sources, would diminish this barrier for smaller hospitals; technological transfer, or assistance in understanding and implementing telemedicine, could reduce the barrier of knowledge about the technology. Such targeted initiatives could potentially improve the ability of small hospitals to finance and deploy telemedicine technologies, better fulfilling the mission of many of the telemedicine grant programs.

The fact that small, rural hospitals were not adopting telemedicine at the rate of their urban counterparts is typical of the burden rural areas have persistently faced in virtually all matters of economic development (Office of Technology Assessment 1991). Without a critical mass of resources—financial, technical, and human—small, rural communities and their hospitals cannot compete in the marketplace, nor can they compete effectively for government programs designed specifically to help them. This research provides more evidence that policy makers need to pay special attention not only to the symptoms of rural distress, but also to its causes.

8.2.2 Ownership status

The profound difference in patterns of telemedicine adoption between not-for-profit (NFP) and (IO) investor-owned hospitals signals the existence of public benefits that make telemedicine an unattractive investment for hospitals whose single objective is to maximize profit. Nonetheless, this finding alone does not prove the existance of public benefits from telemedicine adoption. Policy makers need to understand alternative explanations as to why NFP hospitals are much more likely to adopt telemedicine, and the policy implications of this fact. If the broader mission of NFP hospitals and/or their greater access to grant monies explain this phenomenon, does that mean that telemedicine technologies create a diffuse benefit that is not internalizable as reduced costs or improved revenues? If so, these technologies may be unattractive investments for IO hospitals. In this scenario, the role for government involvement with telemedicine could extend beyond funding start-up costs. If telemedicine has public-good characteristics, there is ample precedent for the role of government. However, if these diffuse benefits, or externalities, do not explain the greater rate of NFP adoption, then future government involvement with this technology may become unnecessary as the technologies become better established and more profitable. More research about the financial, medical, and community benefits of telemedicine is necessary to answer this question. It is important also to discover whether IO hospitals are simply waiting for barriers, such as cost, lack of reimbursement, lack of standards, and lack of physician acceptance, to fall before adopting telemedicine. Perhaps IO hospitals are allowing NFP hospitals to experiment with the technologies and work out some of these difficulties. In this case, the government's role could be seen as temporary, fostering innovation then allowing the internalizable benefits of the technologies to sustain telemedicine development. Many of these questions and scenarios are suggested by this study, but further investigation and more experience with the technologies are necessary to make sound conclusions.

8.2.3   **Strategic role of telemedicine**

This research suggests that telemedicine plays an important role in the competitive strategies of hospitals. For many adopters, telemedicine clearly functions as a marketing tool or form of nonprice competition. Most administrators envision telemedicine to be an important component of their managed care strategy that will increase their market share and enhance patient management and, consequently, reduce costs. These findings point to characteristics of telemedicine that resemble private goods, with internalizable benefits.

If telemedicine becomes an important tool for minimizing costs in a managed care environment, the current debate as to whether the Health Care Financing Administration (HCFA) should reimburse for telemedical consultations could become moot. As one administrator stated, "managed care may be just the ticket for telemedicine." In other words, administrators currently hesitant to implement these technologies without third-party insurance reimbursement would readily use telemedicine if the technology enhanced patient management in a managed care environment.

Although the existence of actual and expected internalizable benefits from telemedicine provides little justification for government involvement, these private benefits do not rule out a role for government. If telemedicine improves the quality of health care in rural areas, allows rural hospitals to remain accredited and in operation, or plays a role in the economic development of a rural community, the argument could be made that the public benefits created by these technologies justify government involvement. This involvement is particularly justified if small and/or rural hospitals are unable to realize the internalizable benefits that telemedicine may confer without federal or state assistance. Again, more research is necessary to establish the magnitude of these types of internalizable benefits relative to the more diffuse externalities these technologies offer. It is a very important finding, however, that these internalizable benefits exist and are expected by hospital administrators in the future as managed care evolves.

8.2.4 Affiliations

In this study, the commonsense notion that hospitals with affiliation relationships are more likely to adopt telemedicine was empirically demonstrated. The association between affiliation and adoption is important for three reasons: (1) The finding encourages policy makers to improve the reach of telemedicine to smaller hospitals and to establish the types of linkages between hospitals that enable telemedicine to make practical sense. Policy makers can qualify grant awards to encourage networking between large and smaller hospitals and to encourage the participation of small hospitals in affiliation arrangements. (2) The finding suggests another strategic role for telemedicine. If the growth of hospital networks is a step along the path to managed care (Cave 1995; Curran and O'Connor 1995; Hospitals and Health Networks 1995; Kripke Byers and Levi-Baumgarten 1995; Nurkin 1995; Shortell, Gillies, and Devers 1995), the fact that network members are twice as likely as nonmembers to adopt telemedicine reinforces telemedicine as an important strategic technology in a competitive hospital marketplace and reinforces the importance of telemedicine in a managed care environment. (3) The finding brings telemedicine into a larger policy debate about affiliations between hospitals. While hospitals and their advocacy organizations argue that affiliations are necessary in a very competitive health care marketplace, the Justice Department, the Federal Trade Commission, and unaffiliated hospitals maintain that these alliances represent anticompetitive activity and potentially violate antitrust laws. To the extent that telemedicine strengthens affiliations, it could play an important role in this debate. Rural hospitals may be at a particular competitive disadvantage without these types of affiliations, raising the possibility that exceptions to antitrust concerns may be appropriate for rural hospitals in order to bolster their financial viability.

8.2.5   Summary of policy implications

Many of the findings of this research help to focus the unanswered questions about telemedicine. Initially, this research identified the lack of financial information about telemedicine, a debilitating limitation to discovering how telemedicine affects the costs of delivering health care.

The lack of financial information calls into question whether telemedicine adopters are able to determine the benefits of the technology in their own institutions. Until more uniform accounting of telemedicine programs within hospitals is available, qualitative research, cost-finding studies, and case-study methods will have to substitute for cross-sectional analyses of the cost effects of telemedicine.

This research also identified a gap between the diffusion of telemedicine and the goals of federal and state policy makers: Telemedicine is not reaching small and rural hospitals. Programs to target these hospitals for technical and financial assistance could improve the access of small hospitals to telemedicine technologies. In addition, the fact that not-for-profit (NFP) hospitals and members of integrated delivery networks (IDNs) are more likely to adopt telemedicine provides information that allows policy makers to use these relationships to better target telemedicine grant programs. In essence, these findings identify key leverage points that policy makers can use to more effectively meet their goals of extending telemedicine technologies into rural communities.

The findings of this study identify a set of questions regarding the types of benefits that telemedicine provides. Are NFP hospitals adopting these technologies out of altruistic commitments to community service with little expectation of internalizing the benefits of telemedicine technologies? Because of their broader mission, are NFP able to experiment with nascent technologies and determine how to make an interesting and seemingly useful technology profitable in the future? As these questions are answered, the role for government in the diffusion of telemedicine technologies will be clarified.

8.3 Importance, limitations, and future directions of this research

This research represents the first cross-sectional empirical study of economic and management aspects of telemedicine adoption. As such, it identifies as many questions as it answers. Nonetheless, important policy implications are derived from the findings of this study. With these results, policy makers can better identify the types of hospitals adopting telemedicine, compare this to their program objectives, and make appropriate improvements to their programs. This research also helps to transform the many questions about telemedicine, suggested in chapters 1 and 2, into a more focused set of inquiries.

In addition to uncovering particular issues of telemedicine and hospitals, this study also highlights issues of perennial concern to rural communities and policy makers concerned with rural issues. Rural areas are often ill suited to attract or compete for many of the resources that would benefit them specifically. Concern about the lack of economic opportunities in rural areas is not new, but this study provides a current example of this phenomenon.

Although this study examines hospitals within the southeastern region of the United States, the limitations in its generalizability are minimal. The parameters of hospital size, ownership structure, and hospital affiliations are not unique to this region. Moreover, with the exception of the west coast and selected cities in the northeast, most of the United States faces health care markets that share a similar evolution to managed care as found in North Carolina, South Carolina, and Georgia. As many states are in early stages of planning their telecommunications policy, the three states studied for this research can serve as an example of what to expect in telemedicine diffusion.

In many ways, this study is limited by the quality of the data obtained through the survey. One of the most important findings from this research—that financial data are virtually nonexistent and certainly inaccessible on a large scale—is also the Achilles' heel of this project. While it is essential from a policy perspective to draw attention to the lack of cost data, which makes cost-benefit calculations and inferences about public welfare impossible, it is also less than satisfying from a research perspective.

The diffusion models specified in this project provided important and policy-relevant information, which will assist policy makers as they fashion and rework policies to support telemedicine. A survey designed specifically for a diffusion model, however, would have provided even more useful information. As described in chapter 4, an ideal diffusion model would differentiate between hospitals that primarily provide telemedicine consultations, those that primarily receive consultations, and those that both provide and receive consultations. Such a model would identify the distinct characteristics of each type of adopter. In doing so, a model could better distinguish and suggest the types of benefits hospitals receive from telemedicine technologies. From an econometric perspective, this would be relatively easily accomplished using a polytomous response-generated logit model. Unfortunately, the questions that would conform to such a model were not sufficiently answered by the respondents to be useful in the type of statistical analysis for this research. If the study had focused on diffusion from the outset, these questions would have been phrased differently and augmented by complementary questions about specific benefits offered by telemedicine technologies.

Alternatively, with the benefit of hindsight, this research could have obtained better cost information if a case-study approach, rather than a survey approach, had been undertaken originally. This was a known risk at the outset of this project. The potential benefit of obtaining cross-sectional financial data from enough hospitals to construct a viable cost model appeared to outweigh the potential cost of failure to do so. A case-study design would have allowed an in-depth exploration of the complex financial arrangements and the real and perceived benefits of these technologies from the perspective of individual hospitals. The telephone and in-person interviews that were conducted as a supplement to the survey proved invaluable in forming an understanding of what the diffusion modeling suggested. Case studies certainly would have improved this level of understanding even more. This approach, however, would not have overcome a fundamental problem with conducting a study of the cost effects of telemedicine at this early stage of its diffusion. As Porter (1980, 217) explains, early costs are not reflective of the true costs of an innovation: "Small production volume and newness usually combine to produce high costs" in the early stages of using a new technology. Since the overwhelming majority of hospitals had adopted telemedicine within the 18 months prior to the survey, this point is particularly relevant.

The limitations of this study are largely a function of the risks of research in general and of the excitement surrounding telemedicine in particular. Because telemedicine has received a great deal of media and policy attention, it seemed an attractive candidate for survey research and was expected to be much more widely diffused at the outset of this project. Only primary data collection could have determined that this was not, in fact, the case. In addition, this study was subject to the same risks as any endeavor involving primary data collection. The survey did not provide adequate data to conduct the research it was intended to inform. As a result, much effort was dedicated to making the best of a less-than-ideal situation. From this perspective, the diffusion model—while not ideal—provides information that is extremely policy relevant and that takes advantage of the available data. The qualitative data provide substantial insight into the relationships suggested by the empirical research. Together, the quantitative and qualitative data represent powerful information for policy makers and an important first for telemedicine research: Nowhere else in the literature to date has cross-sectional information about the adoption of telemedicine appeared.

The many questions raised by this research point to fertile ground for further research. The most obvious next step is a case study–based assessment of hospitals' cost-accounting for telemedicine and an analysis of the impacts of telemedicine on the overall costs for these hospitals. This assessment would involve gaining access to purchasing information, personnel information, and patient information from all telemedicine projects that are active in the selected hospitals. The research would examine how and to what extent the individual hospitals account for telemedicine expenditures and would compare this information to accounting practices for other medical technologies. In many ways, telemedicine is unique due to the extensive government involvement in this area and the lack of reimbursement from traditional sources. A comparison of the similarities and differences between accounting practices across technologies and across hospitals would lay the groundwork for determining the cost-effectiveness of public and hospital investments in telemedicine. Such a comparison would also provide a preliminary framework for accounting for telemedicine across all hospitals and would guide the development of an instrument for systematically collecting this information across all hospitals. With this information, policy makers or researchers could eventually conduct the type of research originally proposed for this study.

Another potential direction for telemedicine research is exploring the nature of the relationships within telemedicine networks. Why are certain hospitals affiliating with each other? Is affiliation an artifact of personal relationships among administrators? Does this alignment depend on prior referral patterns, or are other economic calculations at work? Because antitrust issues have become prominent concerns in the health care marketplace, understanding the implications of the growth and configuration of telemedicine networks in this context is important. This type of research could be conducted effectively with either a survey or case-study approach, each offering its particular strengths and weaknesses.

Another useful direction for further research would increase the generalizability of the findings of this study. With data about telemedicine adoption across general hospitals in other regions of the United States, replicating this study and comparing results across different regions would be possible.

The current study pointed to the need for further research to identify the range of benefits hospitals are deriving from telemedicine technologies to define the appropriate role for government in the evolution of these technologies. Future studies could identify benefits to individual hospitals, to communities, and to patients. As a condition for future federal funding, many telemedicine projects could be polled to document patient satisfaction and medical benefits. These types of benefits will come to light as hospitals gain further experience with telemedicine technologies and construct reports for federal funding agencies.

In summary, this research has provided valuable and policy-relevant information about the diffusion of telemedicine in hospitals in the southeastern United States. The study was conducted at an exciting time in the health care industry, with telemedicine in a state of dynamic and early development. Future diffusion of telemedicine will depend on policies regarding reimbursement, improved identification of costs and benefits, and the vagaries of a "hyper-turbulent" health care market.

NOTES

1. Here, they are paraphrasing David (1986).

2. personal conversation, Steven Downs, program analyst, NTIA, March 15, 1996

3. The figures used for HMO enrollment reflect only enrollment in federally licensed HMOs. This is a subset of all HMOs and thus represents a negative bias relative to actual HMO enrollment. For example, in the Charlotte, Raleigh-Durham, and Greensboro MSAs, enrollment in all HMOs ranges between 23% and 35% of the population (Sheps Center for Health Services Research 1996). These statistics were available only for North Carolina and were not included in the model.

4. The reference to rural areas connotes those regions outside a metropolitan statistical area, as classified by the U.S. Office of Management and Budget.

List of interviewees for survey development

Charles Ayscue, Chief Financial Officer, University of North Carolina Hospitals.

Jeff Blomley, St. Luke's Hospital, Columbus, NC.

Diane Bloom, Project Coordinator, Program on Aging, School of Medicine, University of North Carolina Chapel Hill.

George Brandt, Chief Executive Officer, Martin General Hospital, Williamston, NC.

Alto Byers, Memorial Mission Hospital, Highlands, NC.

Cindy Coker, Chowan Hospital.

Christopher Durrer, Chief Executive Officer, Wilson Memorial Hospital, Wilson, NC.

Helena Feather, Vice President of Medical Information, Trident Regional Hospital, Charleston, SC.

Kevin FitzPatrick, Information Systems Coordinator, Duke University Medical Center.

Charles Frock, Chief Executive Officer, Moore Regional Hospital, Pinehurst, NC.

D. Linda Garcia, Senior Associate, Office of Technology Assessment, U.S. Congress.

James Graham, administrator, Person County Memorial Hospital, Roxboro, NC.

Mary Ruth Green, Chief Financial Officer, Hugh Chatham Memorial Hospital.

Jim Grigsby, Assistant Professor, Health Services Research Center, University of Colorado.

Jim Hague, Vice President, North Carolina Hospital Association.

John E. Hammond, Professor of Pathology and Laboratory Medicine, University of North Carolina Chapel Hill.

Henry Hsiao, Professor of Biomedical Engineering, University of North Carolina, Chapel Hill.

Bob Johnson, Vice President, Operations, Duke University Medical Center.

Dick Jones, Chief Executive Officer, New Hanover Regional Medical Center, Wilmington, NC.

Joe Kapowski, Department of Opthamology, School of Medicine, University of North Carolina, Chapel Hill.

Ed McFall, Chief Information Officer, Pitt County Memorial Hospital.

Terri Olivier, Assistant Director, Regional Services, Institutional Relations Division, University of North Carolina Hospitals.

Tom Ricketts, Director of Rural Research Program, Cecil G. Sheps Center for Health Services Research; Assistant Professor of Health Policy and Administration, School of Public Health, University of North Carolina.

Michael Rose, Carolinas Medical Center.

Ed Rouliski, Technical Director, Bowman-Gray School of Medicine.

Tom Seibert, Professor of Psychiatry, Director of Telemedicine, Director of Continuing Medical Education, Duke University Medical Center.

Rebecca Slifkin, Research Associate, Cecil G. Sheps Center for Health Services Research.

Morgan Tackett, Associate Director, Affiliations—Duke Health Network, Duke University Medical Center.

Mark Williams, Professor of Medicine, Director of the Program on Aging, School of Medicine, University of North Carolina, Chapel Hill.

Bibliography and References Cited

Aldrich JH, Nelson FD. *Linear Probibility, Logit, and Probit Models.* Newbury Park: Sage Publications; 1984.

Alexander J, Lewis BL. The financial characteristics of hospitals rnder for-profit and nonprofit contract management. *Inquiry*, 1984; Fall, 21: 230-242.

American Hospital Association. *AHA Guide to Hospitals in the U.S.* Chicago: American Hospital Association; 1992.

American Hospital Association. *AHA Guide to Hospitals in the U.S.* Chicago: American Hospital Association; 1994.

Anderson J, Sanders J. Developing Georgia's telemedicine network. *Health Care Informatics.* 1993; May 10(5): 66-68.

Arrow, K. Uncertainty and the welfare economics of medical care. *American Economic Review.* 1963; 53: 941-969.

Arthur D. Little, Inc. Telecommunications: Can It Help Solve America's Health Care Problems? July, 1992; Cambridge, MA: Arthur D. Little, Inc.

Austin CJ, Trimm JM. Hospital information systems and strategy: a potential yet to be realized. *Proceedings of the 1992 Annual HIMSS Conference.* Chicago: American Hospital Association; 1992.

Averch L, Johnson. Behavior of the firm under regulatory constraint. *American Economic Review.* 1962; v. 52.

Baldridge J, Victor, Burnham RA.Organizational innovation: individual organizational, and environmental impacts. *Administrative Science Quarterly.* 1975; Vol. 20, June.

Beniger J. *The Control Revolution: Technological and Economic Origins of the Information Society.* Cambridge: Harvard University Press; 1986.

Berg SV, Tschirhart J. *Natural Monopoly Regulation: Principle and Practice,* Cambridge: Cambridge University Press; 1988.

Berki SE. *Hospital Economics*, Lexington, MA: Lexington Books; 1972.

Braeutigam RR, Daughety AF. On the estimation of returns to scale using variable cost functions. *Economic Letters.* 1984; 11: 25-31.

————, Panzar JC. Diversification incentives under 'Price Caps' and 'Cost-Based' regulation. *Rand Journal of Economics.* 1989; v. 20, no.3, Autumn.

Breyer F. The specification of a hospital cost function: a comment on the recent literature. *Journal of Health Economics.* 1987; 6: 147-157.

Brown SJ, Sibley DS. *The Theory of Public Utility Pricing*, Cambridge: Cambridge University Press; 1986.

Calabrese A. The periphery in the center: the information age and the 'Good Life' in rural America. Paper presented for the International Association for Mass Communications Research Conference in Bled, Yugoslavia; 1990.

Carey JW. *Communications as Culture: Essays on Media and Society*, Boston: Unwin Hyman; 1989.

Cave DC. Vertical integration models to prepare health systems for capitation. *Health Care Management Review.* 1995; 20 (1) Winter: 26-39.

Caves DW, Christensen LR, Tretheway MW. Flexible cost functions for multiproduct firms. *Review of Economics and Statistics.* 1980; 62: 477-481.

Coll S. *The Deal of the Century: The Breakup of AT&T*, New York: Simon & Schuster, Inc; 1986.

Cook TD, Campbell DT. *Quasi-Experimentation: Design & Analysis Issues for Field Settings*, Boston: Houghton Mifflin Company; 1979.

Coombs R, Saviotti P, Walsh V. *Economics and Technological Change*, London: Macmillan Education LTD; 1987.

Coopers & Lybrand. How the fittest thrive: providers form affiliations, alliances, and networks. *Prognosis.* Washington, DC: Coopers & Lybrand, L.L.P; October, 1994.

Cowing TG, Holtmann AG. Multiproduct short-run hospital cost functions: empirical evidence and policy implications from cross-section data. *Southern Journal of Economics.* 1983; 49: 637- 653.

Crandall RW, Flamm K, eds. *Changing the Rules: Technological Change, International Competition, and Regulation in Communications*, Washington, DC: The Brookings Institution; 1989.

Curran C, O'Connor DG. Restructuring: a tale of four cities. *Managed Care Quarterly.* 1995; 3 (2): 87-96.

Deaton A, Muellbauer J. *Economics and Consumer Behavior*, Cambridge: Cambridge University Press; 1989.

Deloite & Touche. *New Jersey Telecommunications Infrastructure Study, Vols. 1-3;* January 1991.

Denison E. *Why Growth Rates Differ: Postwar Experience in Nine Western Countries*, Washington, DC: The Brookings Institute; 1967.

Dixon R. Hybrid corn revisited. *Econometrica.* 1980; Vol. 48, No. 6: 1451-1462.

Egan BL, Waverman L. The state of competition in telecommunications. in Barry Cole, ed., *After the Breakup: Assessing the New Post-AT&T Divestiture Era*, New York: Columbia University Press; 1991.

Faulhaber GR, Boyd J. Optimal new-product pricing in regulated industries. *Journal of Regulatory Economics.* 1989; vol. 1: 341-358.

Freshwater D. *Toward Rural Development Policy for the 1990s.* Joint Economic Committee, U.S. Congress, S.Prt. 101-150. Washington, DC: Government Printing Office; 1989.

Friedman B, Shortell S. The financial performance of selected investor-owned and not-for-profit system hospitals before and after medicare prospective payment. *Health Services Research.* 1988; June, 23(2): 237-267.

Gaile GL. The spread-backwash concept. *Regional Studies.* 1980; Vol. 14: 15-25.

Georgia Statewide Academic and Medical System. GSAMS. http://www.gactr.uga.edu/GSAMS/GSAMS.html (March 13, 1996).

Gesler WM, Cromartie J. Studying spatial patterns of illness and hospital use in a Central Harlem health district. *Journal of Geography.* 1985; Volume 84.

Goldberg AJ, DeNoble RA, eds. *Hospital Departmental Profiles*, American Hospital Publishing, Inc.; 1986.

Gormley Jr. WT. *The Politics of Public Utility Regulation*, Pittsburgh, PA: University of Pittsburgh Press; 1983.

Grannemann TW, Brown RS, Pauly MV. Estimating hospital costs. *Journal of Health Economics.* 1986; 5: 107-127.

Grilliches Z. Hybrid corn: an exploration in the economics of technological change. *Econometrica.* 1957; Vol 25, No. 4: 501-522.

———. Hybrid corn revisited: a reply. *Econometrica.* 1980; Vol. 48, No. 6: 1463-1465.

Gujerati DN. *Basic Econometrics, Second Edition*, New York: McGraw-Hill Publishing Company; 1988.

Halpern MT, Alexander JA, Fennell ML. Multihospital system affiliation as a survival strategy for rural hospitals under the prospective payment system. *Journal of Rural Health.* 1992; Vol. 8, No. 2: 93-105.

Hammond JE, Berger, RG, et al. Making the transition from information systems of the 1970s to medical information systems of the 1990s: the role of the physician's workstation. *Journal of Medical Systems.* 1991; Vol. 15, No. 3.

Hansen NM. *Intermediate Size Cities as Growth Centers*, New York: Praeger Publications; 1971.

Hatcher L, Stepanski EJ. *A Step-by-Step Approach to Using the SAS® System for Univariate and Multivariate Statistics*, Cary, NC: SAS Institute; 1994.

Health care Information and Management Systems Society. *Proceedings of the 1992 Annual HIMSS Conference.* Chicago: American Hospital Association; 1992.

Hirschman AO. *The Strategy of Economic Development*, New Haven: Yale University Press; 1958.

Hoerger TJ. 'Profit' variability in for-profit and not-for-profit hospitals. *Journal of Health Economics.* 1991; 10: 259-289.

Homer CG, Bradham DD, Rushefsky M. Investor-owned and not-for-profit hospitals: beyond the cost and revenue debate. Letter in response to Sloan and Vraciu. *Health Affairs.* 1983; 3: 133- 136.

Hospitals & Health Networks. How markets evolve. *Hospitals & Health Networks.* 1995; March 5.

Hospital Product News. EDI would save industry $42 billion, panel concludes. *Hospital Product News.* February 15, 1994: 11.

Innis H. *The Bias of Communication.* Toronto: University of Toronto Press; 1951.

International Telecommunications Union. *Information, Telecommunications, and Development*, Geneva: ITU; 1986.

Isard W. *Methods of Regional Analysis: An Introduction to Regional Science.* Cambridge: MIT Press; 1971.

Jacobs J. *Cities and the Wealth of Nations: Principles of Economic Life.* New York: Vintage Books; 1984.

Joskow P. Inflation and environmental concern: structural change in the process of public utility price regulation. *Journal of Law and Economics.* 1974; Vol. 17.

Kaye RA. Current trends in telecommunications technologies, systems, and services. In Estabrooks MF, Lamarch RH, eds. *Telecommunications: A Strategic Perspective on Regional Economic and Business Development.* Moncton, Canada: The Canadian Institute for Research on Regional Development; 1986.

Keen P. *Competing in Time: Using Telecommunications for Competitive Advantage.* Cambridge, MA: Ballinger Publishing Company; 1986.

Klausen LM, Olsen TE, Risa AE. Technological diffusion in primary health care. *Journal of Health Economics.* 1992; 11: 439-452.

Kralewski J, Gifford G, Porter J. Profit vs. public welfare goals in investor-owned and not-for-profit hospitals. *Hospital and Health Services Administration.* 1988; Fall, 33(3): 311-329.

Kripke-Byers S, Levi-Baumgarten M. Preparing for Health Reform: A Blueprint for Improving Health Care Access, Cost, and Quality in Metropolitan Areas," in *Managed Care Quarterly*. 1993; 3 (2), pp. 77-86.

Landau R, Rosenberg N. *The Positive Sum Strategy: Harnessing Technology for Economic Growth.* Washington, DC: The National Academy Press; 1986.

LaPlante A. A virtual ER. *Forbes ASAP.* 1995; June 5: 49-54.

Lawton R, Borrows J. *Factors Affecting the Definition of the Local Calling Area: An Assessment of Trends.* Columbus, OH: The National Regulatory Research Institute; 1990.

Leff NH. Externalities, information costs and social benefit-cost analysis for economic development: an example from telecommunications. *Economic Development and Cultural Change.* 1984; Vol. 32, No. 2, January.

Lipson LR, Henderson TM. *State Initiatives to Promote Telemedicine.* Primary Care Resource Center, Intergovernmental Health Policy Project. The George Washington University, Washington, DC; 1995.

Machlup F. *The Production and Distribution of Knowledge in the US.* Princeton: Princeton University Press; 1962.

Maddala GS. *Limited-Dependent and Qualitative Variables in Econometrics,* Cambridge: Cambridge University Press; 1994.

McKinney MM, Kaluzny AD, Zuckerman HS. Paths and pacemakers: innovation diffusion networks in multihospital systems and alliances. *Health Care Management Review.* 1991; 16 (1): 17-23.

Microelectronics Center of North Carolina. *Annual Report: Making Technology Work*; 1991.

Mitchell B, Vogelsang I. *Telecommunications Pricing: Theory and Practice.* Cambridge: Cambridge University Press; 1991.

Moscovice I, Johnson J, Finch M, Grogan C, Kralewki J. The structure and characteristics of rural hospital consortia. *Journal of Rural Health.* 1991; Fall: 575-587.

Moss M. Can states face the future? New agenda for telecommunications policy. *New York Affairs.* Special Issue on the State Role in Economic Development. 1986; Vol. 9, No. 3.

Munnell A. Is there a shortfall in public capital investment? An overview. *New England Economic Review.* 1991; May/June.

Mueller D. *Public Choice II*, Cambridge: Cambridge University Press; 1989.

Mueller M. Universal service in telephone history. *Telecommunications Policy.* 1993; July.

Musgrave RA. *Public Finance in a Democratic Society: Volume I*, New York: New York University Press; 1986.

Myrdal G. *Economic Theory and Underdeveloped Regions.* New York: Harper; 1957.

Nadiri I. Producers Theory. in Arrow KJ, Intrilligator MD, eds. *Handbook of Mathematical Economics, Vol. II.* North Holland Publishing Co; 1982.

National Telecommunications and Information Administration. *Telecommunications in the Age of Information,* Washington, DC: Department of Commerce; 1991.

Neuberger N. Commentary: Some Lessons from Experience. In Kaluzny AD, Zuckerman HS, Ricketts, III TC. *Partners for the Dance: Forming Strategic Alliances in Health Care,* Ann Arbor, MI: Health Administration Press; 1995.

New York Times. 150 miles away, the doctor is examining your tonsils. Sept. 16, 1992: C14.

New York Times. Cable company plans a data 'Superhighway. April 12, 1993: C1.

New York Times. US West will buy into Time Warner. May 17, 1993: A1.

New York Times. New wave in health care: visits by video. July 15, 1993: A1.

New York Times. MCI plans to enter local markets. January 5, 1994: C1.

Nicholson W. *Intermediate Microeconomics and its Application,* Chicago: The Dryden Press; 1987.

Noam E. Network tipping and the tragedy of the common network: a theory for the formation and breakdown of public telecommunications systems. Working paper. Columbia Institute for Tele-Informatics. New York: Columbia Graduate School of Business; 1995.

Noll RG. Telecommunications regulation in the 1990s. Working Paper No. 140. Center for Economic Policy Research, Stanford, CA: Stanford University; 1988.

Noll RG, Smart S. The political economics of state responses to divestiture and federal deregulation in telecommunications. Working Paper No. 176. Center for Economic Policy Research, Stanford, CA: Stanford University; 1989.

Nurkin HA. The creation of a multiorganizational health care alliance: the Charlotte-Mecklenburg Hospital Authority. In Kaluzny AD, Zuckerman HS, Ricketts, III TC. *Partners for the Dance: Forming Strategic Alliances in Health Care,* Ann Arbor, MI: Health Administration Press; 1995.

Office of the State Controller. North Carolina's integrated information network. *North Carolina Information Highway.* http://www.ncih.net/nciin/ (March 13, 1996).

Office of Technology Assessment. *Health Care in Rural America,* Washington, DC: OTA-H- 434; 1990.

Office of Technology Assessment. *Rural America at the Crossroads: Networking for the Future*, Washington, DC: OTA-TCT-471; 1991.

Office of Technology Assessment. *Protecting Privacy in Computerized Medical Information*, Washington, DC: OTA-TCT-576; 1993.

Parker EB, Hudson HE, et al. *Electronic Byways: State Policies for Rural Development through Telecommunications*, Boulder, CO: Westview Press; 1992.

Perednia DA, Brown NA. Teledermatology: one application of telemedicine. *Bulletin of the Medical Library Association.* 1995; 83 (1): 42-47.

Pirelli T, Allan J. Two approaches to implementing industrywide EDI. *Medical Product Sales.* 1992; November.

Pred A. The interurban transmission of growth in advanced economies: empirical fFindings versus regional planning assumptions. *Regional Studies.* 1976; Vol. 10.

Raleigh News & Observer. Hunt unveils information network plan. May 11, 1993: 3A.

Richards B. Doctors can diagnose illnesses long distance, to the dispmay of some. *The Wall Street Journal.* January 17, 1996: A1.

Richardson H. *Regional Economics*, New York: Praeger; 1969.

Rogers EM. *Diffusion of Innovations, Third Edition*, New York: The Free Press; 1983.

Romanoff E. The economic base model: a very special case of input-output analysis. *Journal of Regional Science.* 1974; 1: 121-130.

Rose NL, Joskow PL. The diffusion of new technologies: evidence from the electric utility industry. *RAND Journal of Economics.* 1990; Vol. 32, No. 3, Autumn: 354-373.

Rosegger G. *The Economics of Production and Innovation: an Industrial Perspective*, Oxford: Pergamon Press; 1980.

Savitz LA. *The Influence of Maternal Employment on Obstetrical Health Seeking Behavior.* Doctoral Dissertation for the Department of Health Policy and Administration, University of North Carolina, Chapel Hill; 1994.

Scovill KR. *An Introduction to the Regulation of Telecommunications.* Chicago: Telephony Publishing Corporation; 1985.

Sear AM. Compaison of efficiency and profitability of investor-owned multihospital systems with not-for-profit hospitals. *Health Care Management Review.* 1991; 16(2): 31-37.

Shortell SM, Gillies RR, Devers KJ. Reinventing the american hospital. *The Millbank Quarterly.* 1995; Vol. 73, No. 2: 131-160.

Simpson K, Des Harnais S, Jacobs A, Menapace A. Methods for defining medical service areas. In Ricketts, III TC, Savitz LA, Gesler WM, Osborne D.

Geographic Methods for Health Services Research. Lanham, MD: University Press of America; 1994.

Size T. Commentary: some lessons from experience. In Kaluzny AD, Zuckerman HS, Ricketts, III TC. *Partners for the Dance: Forming Strategic Alliances in Health Care*. Ann Arbor, MI: Health Administration Press; 1995.

Sloan FA, Vraciu RA. Investor-owned and not-for-profit hospitals: addressing some issues. *Health Affairs*. 1983; 2: 25-37.

Sloan FA, Jalvona J, Perrin JM, Adamache KW. Diffusion of surgical technology: an exploratory study. *Journal of Health Economics*. 1986; 5: 31-61.

Smits HL, Baum A. Health Care Financing Administration (HCFA) and reimbursement in telemedicine. *Journal of Medical Systems*. 1994; Vol. 19, No. 2: 139-142.

Solow R. Technical change and the aggregate production function. *Review of Economics and Statistics*. 1957; August.

Stein J. *Health Services Research: A Pragmatic Overview*. Chapel Hill, NC: Sheps Center for Health Services Research; 1990.

Stokes ME, Davis CS, Koch GG. *Categorical Data Analysis: Using the SAS© System*. Cary, NC: SAS Institute, Inc.; 1995.

Stoneman P. *The Economic Analysis of Technological Change*. Oxford: Oxford University Press; 1983.

Tarr J. The evolution of the urban infrastructure. In Hanson R, ed. *Perspectives on Urban Infrastructure*. Washington, DC: National Academies Press; 1984.

Tepelensky JD, Pauly MV, Kimberly JR, Hillman AL, Schwartz JS. Hospital adoption of medical technology: an empirical test of alternative models. Working paper. Philadelphia, PA: Leonard Davis Institute of Health Economics, University of Pennsylvania; 1994.

Teske PE. *After Divestiture: The Political Economy of State Telecommunications Regulation*. New York: State University of New York Press; 1990.

Thompson W. Policy-based analysis for local economic development. *Economic Development Quarterly*. 1987; Vol. 1, No. 1, August: 203-213.

U.S. Department of Labor. *Job Descriptions and Organizational Analysis for Hospitals and Related Health Services*. Washington, DC: US Government Printing Office; 1970.

Varian HR. *Microeconomic Analysis, Second Edition*. New York: W.W. Norton & Company; 1984.

Vita MG. Exploring hospital production relationships with flexible functional forms. *Journal of Health Economics*. 1990; 9: 1-21.

Vitaliano DF. On the estimation of hospital cost functions. *Journal of Health Economics*. 1987; 6: 305-318.

Wenders JT. *The Economics of Telecommunications: Theory and Policy.* Cambridge, MA: Ballinger Publishing Company; 1987.

World Health Organization. *Informatics and Telematics in Health: Present and PotentialUses.* Geneva: World Health Organization; 1988.

Wyman G. The maturing of telemedicine technology. *Health Systems Review.* 1994; September/October: 57-62.

Zuckerman HS, Kaluzny AD, Ricketts, III TC. Alliances in health care: what we know, what we think we know, and what we should know. *Health Care Management Review.* 1994; 20 (1): 54- 64.

Index